# The Truth about Breath Tests

# The Truth about Breath Tests

Ronald C. Denney, Ph.D.

NELSON

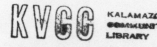

THOMAS NELSON AND SONS LTD
36 Park Street London w1
po Box 2187 Accra
po Box 336 Apapa Lagos
po Box 25012 Nairobi
po Box 21149 Dar es Salaam
77 Coffee Street San Fernando Trinidad

THOMAS NELSON (AUSTRALIA) LTD
597 Little Collins Street Melbourne 3000

THOMAS NELSON AND SONS (SOUTH AFRICA) (PROPRIETARY) LTD
51 Commissioner Street Johannesburg

THOMAS NELSON AND SONS (CANADA) LTD
81 Curlew Drive Don Mills Ontario

First published 1970
Copyright © 1970 Ronald C. Denney

Printed in Great Britain by
Western Printing Services Ltd, Bristol

*This book is dedicated to those people who have encouraged the author in his efforts to convert a collection of data and ideas into a finished work.*

'Our deeds still travel with us from afar,
And what we have been makes us what we are.'   GEORGE ELIOT


'Drink not the third glass – which thou canst not tame
When once it is within thee.'   GEORGE HERBERT


'Who travel to their home among the dead
By the broad highway of the world, and so
With one chained friend, perhaps a jealous foe,
The dreariest and the longest journey go.'
PERCY BYSSHE SHELLEY

# Contents

# Preface

The tremendous increase in the number of cars and drivers on our roads during the past twenty years has led to a corresponding increase in the amount of legislation which exists in attempts to control and restrict the number of road accidents. In recent years, this legislation has taken the form of controls against both unroadworthy vehicles and unroadworthy drivers. As a result, since October 1967 motorists in Great Britain have been subject to a legal maximum limit of the amount of alcohol which they may have in their blood. Prior to this date, such tests had mainly been encountered on the European continent and in the U.S. It is, however, surprising to find that, despite considerable publicity, the average person in this country had, and still has, only a vague idea of what the tests are all about.

It is essential that the layman should have an opportunity to consider the facts behind breath testing and the various methods of determining blood alcohol levels. I have therefore endeavoured to represent chemical and medical data in an easily understood form. This book is not intended for those people who know, or think they know, all the answers, but for those who wish to understand more of the origin and justification of breath tests.

I have attempted to demonstrate the levels of accuracy as well as the limitations which exist in the forms of scientific investigation employed. At the same time, I have considered it essential both to show the effect that alcohol has upon the accident rate and to indicate where the law appears to be badly written. Any criticism is intended to be constructive and is made in the interests of scientific reliability and common justice.

Of necessity the writing of this book has meant crossing the boundaries of several disciplines; while every effort has been made to give correct information and accurate interpretations, I can accept no legal responsibility for any use that may be made of the data contained in this book. Any person charged with driving with more than the prescribed amount of alcohol in his blood is strongly advised to seek full legal advice if he, or she, intends to contest such charges.

The information given in this book is no national secret and has, for the greater part, been obtained from the volumes accessible in such places as the National Reference Library of Science and Invention and the Chemical Society Library. I gratefully acknowledge the additional information that was supplied to me by the Royal Society for the Prevention of Accidents, the Royal Institute of Chemistry, the Automobile Association, the British Medical Association and the American Medical Association.

I wish to thank my former employers, Hopkin & Williams Ltd, for permission to use data collected during the period that I worked for them, and Miss D. Dickson, F.L.A., Acting Chief Librarian of Woolwich Polytechnic, for her considerable efforts in obtaining books and journals from many sources.

I am particularly indebted to Dr E. J. Newman, PH.D., F.R.I.C., to Miss E. Hart, J.P., and to Mr D. Hatwell for spending their time reading the original text and for making constructive suggestions for improvement. My wife, who has assisted with much of the typing, has encouraged me at all stages of writing and has tolerated the long and irregular hours needed to complete the work in a short period of time.

If this book helps to improve the relationship between drivers and police it will have achieved some of its purpose. It is hoped, moreover, that some official attention will be paid to the modifications to the present law that seem so necessary. The use of scientific methods by the police will progressively increase in all realms of law enforcement, and it is essential that the public should have the greatest possible confidence in the equipment employed as well as its method of use. This can only come about if everyone is clearly informed over what is being done both to detect the law-breaker and to protect the law-abiding.

# Introduction

The greater part of the British public was caught completely by surprise when the breath test was introduced into this country, and the initial antagonisms still cloud the attitudes of many people. As there was plenty of advance publicity and discussion about the tests, it is difficult to understand why so little notice was taken until the deadline was reached. It would be fair to say, however, that the British have a built-in blind eye that they turn to all forms of public notices, be they proposed laws, restrictions, take-overs or compulsory purchase orders. This leads to the inevitable claims of 'We didn't know', or the more outraged 'Why weren't we told in advance?' when enforcement actually takes place. When the first breath tests were being applied, this habit took the form of considerable talk about infringing the rights of free citizens, claims that the brewers and publicans would go bankrupt and that the police were carrying out tests indiscriminately.

Much of this emotion arose because the average driver was, and still is, almost completely uninformed about the true scientific basis of the breath test and how it is related to the amount of alcohol in the blood or urine. He is, therefore, naturally suspicious of the scientist and the physician for aiding and abetting the law in adding to the number of restrictions ranged against the motorist. Because of this, there is a tendency for a charged motorist to refuse to acknowledge his responsibility under the law and to seek for some obscure loophole instead of accepting it as an attempt to reduce accidents.

Most people only have access to the rather limited information available in newspaper articles, plus the often apparently conflicting evidence of experts in the law reports. The purpose of this book is to inform the public about the full nature of breath tests, how they have grown up, the chemical basis for the tests, and the level of accuracy that can be expected from determinations carried out on blood and urine. It should be added that through writing this book the author has found himself in complete agreement with the idea of using what has become known in this country as the 'Breathalyser', and in establishing a legal maximum for blood alcohol for road users. He believes that this attempt to reduce road accidents would command much greater respect and co-operation from the driving public if they knew a little more about the facts.

There are more old wives' tales and mistaken concepts about drinking and driving than about practically any other every-day activity. The hardened drinker will always claim that he drives better after two or three pints than he did before, and conversely the teetotaller will continue to believe that a half-pint late at night makes you unfit to drive the following day. Many of these claims and fallacies are answered in the following chapters; only the most prejudiced person will dismiss the evidence as irrelevant. It should be borne in mind that the vast majority of motorists at some time drive when they have a measurable amount of alcohol in their blood. If it is not the government's intention to ban drinking prior to driving com-pletely, it is essential for some guidance to be given to people who have no wish to be a danger on the road but who would still like to know how far they can go in sharing in any festivi-ties. An attempt is made in this book to supply this information based upon reliable sources.

The responsible motorist will always co-operate with any reasonable approach to reducing accidents if he is convinced of its value and purpose. This can only be achieved if he is told what it is all about in as straightforward a manner as possible.

The author has tried to produce a book that will be of interest and value to every driver, particularly those who are convinced that it is safe to drive after drinking several pints of the local 'best'. Scientific and medical researches are con-tinually adding to our knowledge concerning alcohol and accidents. In such an expanding field there still exists a number of controversial points that need to be clarified before the present law can be adequately rewritten and strengthened.

Throughout the book the word 'alcohol' is employed to mean the active constituent of intoxicating liquors. On occa-sions, where appropriate, the more correct chemical names of 'ethyl alcohol' or 'ethanol' are used to differentiate between this and related chemical substances.

# CHAPTER ONE

# Alcohol Through the Years

The effect that alcohol has upon the nervous system is something which has been well known since man first found that the fermentation of plant matter could give rise to liquids which created a euphoric state of mind and enabled him to escape temporarily from the world around him. It is generally accepted that, in all probability, alcohol was the first pain-killer to be used for tooth extractions and primitive operations. Certainly, even the most primitive of tribes on this planet appear to have developed their own brands of 'fire-water' or 'mountain dew' to employ on ceremonial occasions, often to overcome normal inhibitions.

Solomon with all his wisdom was fully conscious of the dangers of excessive drinking and expressed himself pungently on the subject: 'Wine is a mocker, strong drink is raging and whosoever is despised thereby is not wise.' Shakespeare, however, usually seems to take a more liberal attitude to drinking in all its forms, whether towards the hale and hearty consumption by Falstaff and his friends in *Henry IV* or the excesses of the porter in *Macbeth*; the latter being more conscious of both the advantages and disadvantages of consuming large quantities of ale.

Because of the social problems associated with alcohol, it is normal for it to be included under the general heading 'drugs' and is sometimes mentioned in books dealing with drugs and their associated problems. It is generally regarded as occupying an intermediate position between addiction-forming and habit-forming drugs.

Throughout the centuries, alcoholic liquors have always had their opponents as well as their protagonists, and periods of licence have often been followed by prohibition, as in the U.S.

in 1920, the excesses of the few being the excuse to deny enjoyment and relaxation to the majority. Fortunately, most countries are now passing through a more enlightened period where alcohol, taken in moderation and under the right circumstances, is socially acceptable. At the same time, there are still many people who fail to establish a balance between their personal enjoyment and their responsibilities within the community. Because of this, many laws being introduced throughout the world are concerned with preventing alcohol from being the cause of unnecessary accidents without prohibiting its social uses.

Until the end of the seventeenth century, the chief form of alcoholic liquor in Britain was beer, and the licensing of drinking houses, similar to the system existing today, was introduced in 1688 to control its consumption. The Act did not apply to spirits and led to the vast increase in spirit sales, especially gin, during the early eighteenth century. The only attempt to impose what was virtually prohibition of spirits came in 1736, when a tax of 2s. 6d. a pint was imposed on all spirits. This Act only remained in force for seven years, and since then the sales of spirits and beer have been treated in the same way and no attempt at prohibition has been successful. Little attention was paid to the distorting effects that alcohol has upon a person's responses until the advent of the motor vehicle late in the nineteenth century, since when Parliament has progressively tightened up on the motorist with Acts of Parliament designed to discourage people from combining drinking and driving. The first Act of this kind, the Licensing Act of 1872, applied only to carriages, horses, cattle and steam engines; while the first vehicle to be propelled by an internal combustion engine had been built by Karl Benz as early as 1885, their development in England was until 1896 severely impeded by strict legislation aimed at protecting pedestrians and horse-drawn carriages. Not until the Criminal Justice Act 1925 did it become an offence to be found 'drunk in charge of any mechanically driven vehicle'; although the lack of a definition for the word 'drunk' made interpreting the law very difficult. Five years later, the Road Traffic Act 1930 rephrased the offence as being 'under the influence of drink or a drug to such an extent as to be incapable of having proper control of a vehicle', in the hope of making the law tighter and easier to apply. But this, in its turn, suffered from many deficiencies which lasted until the Road Traffic Act 1962 in which the offence was referred to as 'the ability to drive properly is for the time being impaired'. This recognized for the first time that it is not necessary for a person to be incapable of driving for him to become a danger owing to the influence of alcohol. Despite the advent of the later Road Safety Act 1967, which imposed the 80 mg. of alcohol per 100 ml. blood limit, the earlier 1962 Act remains in force. Thus a person with a blood alcohol level below the 80 mg. limit *can* be charged if it can be shown that his driving ability has been impaired through taking alcohol or other drugs.

During the past hundred years numerous attempts have been made to place the study of drinking and its effects on a more objective and scientific basis. That this is still not perfect is obvious from the number of successful appeals which have been made against convictions for drunken driving and related charges.

Although chemical tests to show alcohol concentrations in body tissues have been available for a hundred years, until October 1967 an accused motorist in this country could stand or fall by the subjective observations of a medical practitioner, who was probably half asleep through having been woken up in the middle of the night. The difficulties of proving intoxication on the basis of a limited physical examination became obvious to the British Medical Association at a very early stage, and a committee set up by its Council produced its first report, *Tests for Drunkenness*, as early as 1927. This report, with later modifications, was used as the criterion for the various examinations carried out on inebriated drivers in police stations. It included various tests involving walking in a set direction, showing an ability to write and to add or subtract.

While we, in Britain, were busy setting up the first of many committees, the first determination of blood alcohol on the basis of a sample of exhaled breath was carried out in the U.S. This pioneering work, by Dr Bogen, led to the development of portable forms of apparatus that could easily be operated by police in carrying out on-the-spot tests. The first successful apparatus, patented in 1938, put the U.S. far ahead in the field of investigating drunken driving. Since then several other on-the-spot apparatuses have been developed for both

qualitative (screening) and quantitative (conclusive) testing.
The result of this has been that, in most states of the U.S., it is
possible to be convicted of 'driving under the influence of
intoxicating liquor' simply on the result of a breath test carried
out at the roadside. The rather complicated apparatus employed to do this is intended to give an almost instantaneous
reading of the blood alcohol level based upon the breath
alcohol content.

While the Americans were busy inventing breath-testing
machines and passing state laws in attempts to reduce the ever-
rising numbers of injured and dead on the roads, the British
Medical Association was still trying to make people aware of
the fact that it is not necessary for a driver to be blind drunk
for him (or her) to be incapable of adequately controlling a
motor vehicle. In 1960, a special committee of the B.M.A.
produced a report entitled *Relation of Alcohol to Road
Accidents*, which said among its conclusions:

> The Committee considers that a concentration of 50 mg. of
> alcohol in 100 ml.* of blood while driving a motor vehicle is
> the highest that can be accepted as entirely consistent with the
> safety of other road users. While there may be circumstances in
> which individual driving ability will not depreciate signifi-
> cantly by the time this level is reached, the Committee is
> impressed by the rapidity with which deterioration occurs at
> blood levels in excess of 100 mg./100 ml. This is true even in
> the case of hardened drinkers and experienced drivers. The
> Committee cannot conceive of any circumstances in which it
> could be considered safe for a person to drive a motor vehicle
> on the public roads with an amount of alcohol in the blood
> greater than 150 mg./100 ml.

It should be pointed out that these figures had similarly been
arrived at in 1938 by a committee of the National Safety
Council in the U.S. and formed the basis for much of the early
legislation concerned with drinking and driving in that country.

* Metric quantities are employed throughout this book as results, and
values are normally expressed in this manner:
1 mg. (milligramme) = 1/1,000 gm. (gramme)
28·3 gm. = 1 ounce
100 ml. (millilitres) = 0.1 litre = 0.18 pint

The first real step in Great Britain towards the introduction of scientific methods for determining the quantity of alcohol in a driver's blood was actually the Road Traffic Act of 1962. This particular Act did not make it compulsory for an accused motorist to supply a sample of blood or urine when asked to do so by a police constable, but it did establish that refusal to consent to provide a sample could be used as supporting evidence for the prosecution concerning his condition at the time. The procedures to be followed in obtaining, dividing, supplying and analysing the specimens of blood or urine were laid down, and are those currently applied. It is not usually realized that the 1962 Act contains the first mention of the possibility of police asking for breath samples for analysis. At that time no figures for the relationship between alcohol in blood, urine and breath had been defined and no apparatus for taking breath samples approved.

As a result of more committees, further studies and additional reports, the government eventually felt that the road accident figures were severe enough to justify tighter restrictions against drinking and driving. The Road Safety Act of 1967, introduced by Mrs Barbara Castle, then Minister of Transport, was actually more devoted to controls on goods vehicles than anything else. It will, however, be primarily remembered for the eight pages in which the breath tests and their associated penalties are detailed.

The 1967 Act does not define the form of apparatus that the police may employ to carry out the test, since the Home Office is free to recommend the use of any apparatus which meets its standards. At present only one form of device has been approved, this being the apparatus known colloquially as the 'Breathalyser', but supplied under the registered trade mark of 'Alcotest 80' by Draeger Normalair Ltd of Blyth, Northumberland. This apparatus, described in detail in Chapter 4, as well as any other likely to be approved by the Home Secretary in the future, is only intended under the terms of the 1967 Act to be used for screening purposes. It is not intended that any prosecution should be brought on the basis of a positive result from a breath test. Such a result can be used only as a justification for the police to demand a blood or urine sample for further quantitative study. Further proceedings can then only be taken if the chemical tests on these samples indicate an alcohol content in the blood above the prescribed limit of 80 mg./100 ml.

The 80 mg. limit appears to be a compromise between advocates of a 50 mg. limit and those favouring a higher 100 mg. limit. This could be termed a typical British approach to the problem, as it places us in a small group occupied only by Northern Ireland, Austria and four of the states of the U.S., and suggests that at some time in the future the limit could be lowered to the more restrictive 50 mg. level. Although Northern Ireland is part of the United Kingdom, the Stormont government has been responsible for its own legislation on drinking and driving. While they have followed Great Britain in adopting the 80 mg. limit, they have chosen to use a more sophisticated machine which gives automatic blood readings from breath samples in roadside breath tests.

Foreign countries have paid closer attention to the various medical reports in establishing blood alcohol limits. The fifty U.S. states have all been responsible for their own legislation, but, with the exception of the four states already mentioned, have chosen the higher levels of either 100 or 150 mg. as adequate evidence of driving under the influence. In most European countries where legal limits have been adopted, the accepted levels vary from 150 mg. in the case of Belgium to 50 mg. in Norway and Sweden. The lowest limit appears to be that imposed by Czechoslovakia, where, although no maximum limit is written into legislation, drivers are prohibited by law from drinking before or during driving. In practice, only drivers with a blood alcohol level above 30 mg./100 ml. are charged with breaking the law.

In discussing the recommended figures for acceptable blood alcohol levels, it should be borne in mind that they are *not* arbitrary levels arrived at by doddering theoreticians gathered around a lucky-dip tub. They represent conclusions reached from physiological studies on the effects of alcohol on the central nervous system which have been carried out with increasing frequency since the turn of the century. Over the years this has led to the accumulation of a considerable amount of data on people's responses after drinking alcoholic beverages. Every conceivable form of test has been carried out to investigate co-ordination and reaction times in people who have consumed different quantities of alcohol under various conditions. The tests employed have ranged from simple finger-to-finger touching exercises to the more involved use of construction sets, written examinations and complex traffic simulators. Even the most elementary of these tests have given results to support the general conclusion that, the greater the level of blood alcohol, the slower the speed of reaction in an emergency.

It is accepted by the medical profession that the effect of alcohol leads to a progressive deterioration of co-ordination. The idea that a very small quantity of alcohol can actually lead to an improvement in a driver's response has been wholly discredited, measurable deterioration having been observed in subjects with only a 10 mg. blood alcohol level. Dr M. Hebble-linck, in Belgium, has shown that people with blood alcohol levels as low as 30 mg./100 ml. exhibit greatly decreased posture control and a reduction in physical power. Similar studies throughout the world substantiate the view that, at no stage, does alcohol lead to improvement in driving ability or general self-control. Also contrary to popular belief, the reaction time and co-ordination tests reveal no great variation between different individuals, be they abstainers or hardened drinkers; though the latter group is probably better at hiding the effects of drinking when it comes to talking and general demeanour.

Up to the 50 mg. level, impairment of co-ordination, while measurable by response tests, is unlikely to be observable to the casual onlooker. Above this level, progressive impairment is noticeable even without resorting to tests, and this is the reason why the 50 mg. level is accepted by many countries as being the starting-point for prosecution. Above 100 mg., deterioration of responses in the various co-ordination tests occurs rapidly and is the reason why this level has been accepted as suitable for prosecution by rather more liberal legislators. It is difficult to understand how a legislative body genuinely concerned with reducing the number of road accidents can justify the use of the 150 mg. level as a minimum to warrant prosecution. The response tests show that, between the 100 and 150 mg. levels, impairment is so serious that any driver with this amount of alcohol in his system is highly accident prone; as is shown by the figures given on page 19.

Although drinking is usually mentioned in its relation to driving, observations on impairment of response and co-ordination apply equally to other forms of transport and machinery. The heavy drinker is as much a danger on a bicycle or operating a circular saw as he would be driving a car.

As with traffic lights and speed restrictions, the breath test and the 80 mg. blood alcohol limit are added infringements on our rights and freedoms. They have, however, been imposed in the interests of the community as a whole. Rights and freedoms only extend so far as they do not interfere with the corresponding rights of others. To enjoy the privilege of driving a piece of machinery weighing several hundredweight at high speed along the roads, we must be prepared to forgo the right simultaneously to imbibe a large quantity of alcoholic liquor. The objective behind the breath test is a perfectly laudable one, but needs to be appreciated for what it is – a relatively simple chemical screening test that determines whether or not a person has an amount of alcohol in his system that is near or above the legal maximum. It is the later blood, or urine, analysis which establishes whether or not the legal limit has been exceeded.

# CHAPTER TWO

# Alcohol in Breath, Blood and Urine

As we have seen, over a period of many years numerous studies have been carried out to ascertain the relationship between the amount of alcohol found in the various tissues and organs of individuals who have consumed varying quantities of alcoholic beverages and their responses. As most drinkers will be aware, however, the effect of alcohol is not necessarily instantaneous, and therefore any studies must take into consideration the time which has elapsed since a drink was taken by the subject under examination.

The greatest concentrations of alcohol arise in those body tissues which possess the greatest proportions of water. As the brain has a very high water content, it is not surprising that alcohol starts to affect the central nervous system within a matter of minutes after being consumed. The rapid transfer of alcohol to the body fluids is well known to nursing mothers who breast feed their infants. Alcohol from half a pint of beer or a glass of gin will pass into the body milk within five to ten minutes, and in this way acts as a soporific for a crying or fretting baby.

The rate of absorption of alcohol is dependent upon the amount consumed and whether or not it is taken into an empty stomach. It may be over an hour before the alcohol is completely absorbed and passing round the human system by transfer between tissue, blood and urine. Alcohol taken with a meal or on a full stomach is definitely absorbed more slowly than that taken on an empty stomach. This is owing both to the alcohol being diluted by the stomach contents, and to the fact that food components tend to line the stomach and delay its absorption. In the early stages, alcohol is absorbed into the body tissues more quickly than it can be burnt up or eliminated. This leads to the blood alcohol level rising over a period of time to a maximum figure between thirty to sixty minutes after alcohol consumption has ceased. After the maximum is reached, the level falls at a fairly constant rate until all the alcohol has been destroyed within the body or passed into the urine.

At the same time, the distribution of alcohol between various body tissues reaches an equilibrium about an hour after consumption ceases. This equilibrium, of a progressively decreasing amount of alcohol, is maintained until it has all been eliminated. After a delay of one hour, it is possible to determine the alcohol content of almost any part of the body by analysis of a sample taken from it. Thus an accurate measure of alcohol in the urine can be related to a corresponding value for blood and a similar value for breath.

As a result of much investigation, it is accepted, for the basis of tests in Great Britain, that urine contains about 1·33 times the amount of alcohol as does an equal volume of venous blood taken from the same subject at the same time. Because of this, the Road Safety Act of 1967 considers that a urine sample showing an alcohol content of 107 mg./100 ml. is comparable with a blood sample giving a result of 80 mg./100 ml.

The reason why this relationship can be extended to breath is because there is a constant interchange between any alcohol in the blood and the air in a person's lungs. Therefore, anybody who has been drinking will continuously exhale a small quantity of alcohol with his breath as long as there is any remaining in his blood stream. A volume of exhaled breath from the depth of the lungs will contain 1/2,100 of the amount of alcohol as an identical volume of blood. As a result, the extent of the chemical reaction given by the breath sample can be related within well-established limits to the alcohol in the blood.

Having considered the relationship between the alcohol ratios, however, it is necessary to draw attention to possible discrepancies and sources of error that can occur between them.

Alcohol is absorbed into the blood stream rapidly after consumption, but is not observed in the urine for a period of time which varies between fifteen and thirty minutes. During this time samples of the two fluids will bear no relationship to each other. No constant balance between the body fluids can be attained while alcohol is still being consumed, so that the blood alcohol figure will, during consumption, be higher than the urine alcohol figure (allowing for the 1·33 ratio). It is not until at least 30 minutes after the final quantity of alcohol has been consumed that the figures for blood alcohol and urine alcohol are at all comparable; and only then if the bladder has been previously emptied. If the drinker's bladder has not been emptied prior to, or during, the course of the drinking session, a sample of urine taken for analysis is likely to give a low alcohol figure. This difficulty is overcome by discarding the first sample of urine and taking a second sample about half an hour later to use for the analysis. It would, however, be fair to say that urine samples are only fully accurate if the drinker has emptied his bladder at frequent intervals during the course of his drinking session.

As the breath alcohol content arises from the direct interchange with the blood in the capillaries of the lungs, it is possible for this to be a far more accurate measure of the alcohol content of the blood while a person is still drinking and immediately after he has stopped drinking. The current breath test device employed in Britain is not accurate enough for conclusive measurements of this type, but most of the instruments operated in the U.S. are, and have been used to obtain results later presented as evidence in court proceedings.

Even the use of blood samples for establishing a legal limit has met with some opposition as the alcohol content can vary depending upon whether it is taken from the arteries, the veins or the capillaries. This variation occurs mainly during the time that alcohol is being continuously consumed and tends to level out rapidly after drinking has ceased. By the time samples are taken for chemical analysis, the equilibrium state will have been reached so that this temporary variation does not invalidate the tests.

Professor Payne and his colleagues at the Royal College of Surgeons have drawn attention to discrepancies existing in the alcohol content of venous and capillary blood samples taken from volunteers who have consumed various quantities of alcoholic liquor. They found that alcohol is not evenly distributed between the plasma (the liquid part of the blood) and the red blood cells (the solid part of the blood), so that the plasma tends to show a higher alcohol content than do the red blood cells or the blood sample as a whole. As the alcohol content of breath is dependent upon the alcohol content of the blood plasma in the capillaries rather than that of the blood cells, they have suggested that alcohol in blood plasma figures should be used in place of the present figures for complete blood. This would mean re-expressing the 80 mg./100 ml. value for complete blood as 95 mg./100 ml. if plasma alone is used, as the alcohol ratio between the two is 1 : 1·18.

One of the amusing side-lights of the imposition of breath tests has been the sight of slightly inebriated people doing physical jerks and running round the block in an effort to wear off the effects of the alcohol they have consumed. The only likely result of this exercise, usually taken late at night, is to be arrested either as a suspect person or for being drunk and disorderly. Similarly, drinking copious draughts of black coffee is not likely to reduce the quantity of any alcohol that has already been drunk and absorbed into the circulatory system.

The elimination of alcohol from the system occurs mainly by destruction within the body. Oxygen from air in the lungs converts the alcohol through various chemical stages until it can be exhaled in the form of carbon dioxide.* Water, which is also formed by the metabolic processes, is passed out with the urine. About 90 per cent of the alcohol in the body is used up in this way, and the rate of conversion is not likely to be increased by any noticeable extent as the result of a little short-term exercise. It would require some extensive form of activity such as a long-distance race to remove any substantial amount of alcohol. The remaining 10 per cent of the alcohol consumed is eliminated from the body in an unchanged form in urine, breath and perspiration, the greater proportion of this passing out in the urine.

It is unlikely that the human system is ever completely free from alcohol, even after total abstinence from intoxicating liquors. Numerous investigators have shown the presence of small quantities of alcohol within the range 1–4 mg./100 ml. in blood samples taken from temperate subjects.

Different people of various shapes and sizes eliminate alcohol

* The nature of the chemical process is explained in more detail in Appendix A.

at different rates, and it is only possible to give approximate values as a guide to the decrease of alcohol in the human body after drinking has ceased. Because of this, it has become general to take as a reference point the rate of elimination from the average man weighing 150 lb. Various authorities consider that such a person is capable of eliminating something between 6 and 10 grammes of alcohol in an hour. Such a wide range of values arises from the fact that habitual drinkers are apparently capable of eliminating alcohol more rapidly than abstainers. The conditioned drinker will, therefore, tend to recover far more quickly from the effects of drinking compared with the infrequent drinker.

On the basis of the number of mg. alcohol/100 ml. blood, this can be interpreted to mean that the average individual eliminates between 10 to 15 per cent of his body alcohol in any single hour. So a person with a 100 mg. level of alcohol in his blood at the time he stops drinking, will be down to 85–90 mg. within an hour. Such a rate of burn-up obviously works to the advantage of anybody who is a marginal suspect at the time the breath test is taken, as he is very likely to be below the limit by the time a blood sample has been removed. Conversely, anyone giving a blood sample that has more than 80 mg. alcohol/100 ml. when analysed was in all probability well above that level at the time the breath test was applied.

One other factor that should be borne in mind is that anyone reaching a 200 mg. or higher level during an evening's drinking which finishes at midnight or later, is quite likely to have a blood alcohol level above 80 mg. still remaining by the following morning when he drives to work. It is because of this that successful prosecutions have taken place of people who have not been drinking for several hours. As it is possible to reach a blood alcohol level of about 600 mg./100 ml. before the concentration is great enough to kill, this indicates that a really heavy drinker could be above the legal limit for as long as a day and a half after his last drink.

In a publication entitled *Recognition of Intoxication*, published in 1954, the British Medical Association included a table converting the values for blood alcohol into the corresponding numbers of pints of beer or measures of whisky consumed that would be the minimum possible to give that particular value. This table was later considered to be unreliable, as the level of alcohol depends upon the circumstances under which it was consumed. Because of this it was omitted from the later B.M.A. publication, *The Drinking Driver*, in 1965.

At present it is fair to say that neither the B.M.A. nor the Ministry of Transport is prepared to give any form of a guide to drinkers as to when they are likely to go over the limit. This has been justified on the basis of 'If you drink, don't drive', and is by far the best policy. By choosing a specific blood alcohol level for the purposes of law enforcement, there is an automatic implication, however unintentional, that below this level it is safe to drive and above this level dangerous. It is often pointed out that the very imposition of a statutory limit can encourage motorists to drink to the limit and lead to an increase in accidents arising as a result of drink. Because of this, some guidance needs to be given for the benefit of the more responsible drivers who have no wish to become menaces on the road. Failure to do this ignores the possibility that a person who has not been drinking heavily and does not know where he stands relative to the legal limit, is quite likely to be easily persuaded to take 'one for the road' because he has a false idea of what is required to exceed the limit.

The following figures, compiled on the basis of several sources, are only intended as a rough guide. Allowance must always be made for the circumstances under which drinking has taken place and the period of time over which it has been spread. The basis for most figures being the average 150 lb. man, the same amount of alcohol in a lighter man leads to a higher blood alcohol level, and in a heavier person to a lower level. It is possible to deduct 10 mg. from the level for every hour that has passed since drinking started.

Four whiskies (two doubles), or two pints of beer taken within a short period of time, will lead to a 90 mg. blood alcohol level within about thirty minutes. The *British Medical Journal*, at the time the breath test was introduced, advised drivers who felt it impossible to avoid drinking to stick to the 'Rule of three' – three single measures of whisky or three half-pints of beer. The fastest rate of continuous drinking for a period of seven hours works out as one whisky or one half-pint of beer every hour; equivalent to three and a half pints of beer from start to finish before the limit is reached. This is possible because of the elimination of alcohol that occurs simultaneously with the drinking. It must be emphasized that drinking at a faster rate than this will lead to the limit being attained in a shorter period and with fewer drinks. These figures are based upon the assumption that little or no solid food has been taken with the drinks. Where a good meal is eaten during the course of drinking, experiments confirm that, as this leads to the alcohol being absorbed more slowly into the body, it is possible to drink about four to five single whiskies or halves of beer before reaching the 80 mg. limit.

Comparable figures for wines are not possible as different varieties vary greatly in their alcoholic proportions and as they are usually drunk with fairly substantial meals.

In its original table, the B.M.A. pointed out that in the case of women the legal limit is attained with fewer drinks, and the figures used for the average male need to be reduced by 40 per cent (i.e. to three-fifths of the amount) to be relevant for the average female. It is therefore necessary for women to be even more cautious than men about their drinking, and suggests that it is not necessarily always wise for the drinking husband to allow his apparently more temperate partner to drive the car home.

There is evidence to support the popular belief that a pint of milk drunk before taking alcoholic beverages will help to maintain a low blood alcohol level. Investigations carried out by D. S. Miller and his colleagues at Queen Elizabeth College, London, showed that the milk led to a 50 per cent reduction in the average maximum concentration of blood alcohol. This work was, in fact, used as the background for a large-scale marketing campaign for milk. The experimental figures, however, only applied to subjects in whom the normal maximum blood alcohol level was about 40 mg./100 ml., and are not necessarily applicable to the same extent at higher levels or when a person is likely to be above the legal limit, but these were not investigated.

The value of charcoal/kaolin pills taken before a drinking session is even less certain than that of milk. They are intended to prevent intoxication by coating the lining of the stomach with kaolin to slow down the absorption of the alcohol, while at the same time reducing the amount of free alcohol by the adsorption of some of it on the charcoal. It is unlikely that one small pill will have much effect upon a person who drinks enough to go over the limit, though this is one region where further scientific study could be of value.

Another preparation intended to produce lower blood alcohol levels consists of a mixture of fructose and ascorbic acid (Vitamin C). Some substantiation for the claim has been found in studies in which the mixture led to a lowering of maximum blood alcohol levels by an average of 15 mg. It did not, however, appear to increase the rate at which the alcohol was used up by the body.

None of these commercial preparations have been designed to confuse either the breath or blood tests. Their purpose is to prevent alcohol from entering the blood stream either by absorbing it or by using it up in some other chemical process. Any attempt to market a pill deliberately designed to confuse the tests could be construed as an attempt to obstruct the law.

# CHAPTER THREE

# Alcohol and Accidents

Much of the opposition to breath tests has come from ill-informed people who will not accept that there is any relationship between amounts of blood alcohol and the likelihood of having an accident. These same people are usually the ones who claim that the figures showing a reduction in the number of accidents since the introduction of the tests can be attributed almost entirely to other road safety measures.

The amount of data that has been collated throughout the world concerning the possible relationship between alcohol and accidents is vast. Most of these investigations show that the more alcohol there is in the body, the slower the reaction when an emergency arises. This slowing down of reaction time shows itself in an increase in the accident proneness of a driver which can be directly related to his blood alcohol level.

For many years, the general view was that ethyl alcohol could only be held to account in less than 5 per cent of road accidents. During the past twenty years, a large number of studies in depth have shown that figure to be greatly inaccurate since it reflected only those accidents in which the effect of alcohol was blatantly obvious. These studies, carried out in many countries, have all confirmed that alcohol plays a much greater part than was originally believed. Thus an investigation in Perth, Australia, in 1957 found that of 218 fatal road accident victims, eighty-six (39 per cent) had blood alcohol levels exceeding 100 mg./100 ml. Another study, in Ontario in 1959, showed that drinking drivers were involved in a significantly higher than average number of accidents per year and per mile driven. Similarly, in the U.S., a report was made in 1959 on drivers killed in accidents involving no other vehicle and no other person. The results showed that 69 per

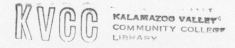

cent of the victims had blood alcohol levels exceeding 50 mg./ 100 ml.

Figures consistent with those published for other countries have been obtained by the Road Research Laboratory in Great Britain. One of their studies, published in 1958, covering three police districts for up to two years, showed that 18 per cent of fatalities arose in accidents in which at least one of the principal parties was known to have consumed alcohol a short time before the accident. More particularly, for accidents occurring between 10 p.m. and 4 a.m., 50 per cent of drivers and 62 per cent of pedestrians had been drinking. Figures closely related to these, covering accidents during 1953 and 1954 in Rutland and Leicestershire, have been published by Dr N. I. Spriggs. He concluded that at least 10 per cent of the fatal road accidents he considered were owing to the intoxication of drivers or pedestrians, and that 50 per cent of the deaths after 10 p.m. could be attributed to this cause.

As early as 1938, research on accidents in Evanston, U.S.A., indicated that a driver with a blood alcohol level of 110 mg./ 100 ml. was seventeen times more likely to be involved in an accident than under normal conditions. A similar study by Professor Vamosi in Bratislava, Czechoslovakia, produced the following figures for accident proneness with increased blood alcohol content:

|  | Accident proneness |
|---|---|
| 30 mg./100 ml. | taken as unity |
| 100 mg./100 ml. | 7 times |
| 150 mg./100 ml. | 30 times |
| Greater than 150 mg./100 ml. | 124 times |

These results are very similar to those obtained in a more detailed survey carried out in Michigan in the United States which covered accidents over a full year (1962) in the city of Grand Rapids. Its purpose was to investigate any relationship between accidents and the nine variables of blood alcohol, age, annual mileage, education, race, marital status, occupation, sex and drinking frequency. To achieve this, 5,985 drivers involved in accidents were interviewed together with 7,590 non-accident drivers. The relationship between blood alcohol content and accidents was based upon 622 accidents in which no other vehicle was involved. Results from this, represented as a graph in Figure 1, take the accident proneness as unity below the 10 mg. level. On this basis, accident proneness is doubled at 60 mg. and rises rapidly to twenty-five times at the 150 mg. level. None of the other eight variables studied showed a relationship of this nature, although they indicated that the most dangerous combination of factors would be a young, drunken driver who was a poorly educated manual worker, still single and only averaging about 1,000 miles a year.

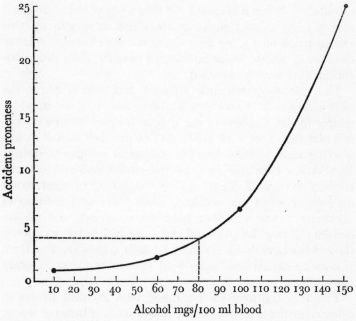

Figure 1. The relationship between accident proneness and blood alcohol content

From the graph, it will be seen that any increase in accident proneness is insignificant until the 50 mg. level has been exceeded. This clearly supports the contention that it is above this level that alcohol can be considered to contribute progressively to road accidents. At the 80 mg. level, accident proneness is four times that for the 10 mg. level.

If the unconvinced require further evidence, it can be pointed out that, apart from the major accident periods which occur during rush-hours, the next peak accident period during any working day occurs between 10 p.m. and midnight. On Saturday evening, the heaviest social and drinking night of the week, the casualty figures for this particular two-hour period are at least as twice as high as for any other two-hour period during the whole week.

Prior to the commencement of breath tests in October 1967, the Royal Society for the Prevention of Accidents (RoSPA) estimated that we could expect a possible reduction of about 5 per cent in the accident figures as a result of their being introduced. When it is considered that 7,319 people were killed and 362,659 injured on the roads of this country in 1967, to talk in terms of a 5 per cent reduction represented 360 fewer deaths and 18,000 fewer injuries. In practice, these prognostications were greatly exceeded.

Unfortunately, very little attention has been drawn to the tremendous cost of accidents to the nation. It is not simply a matter of car damage or the cost of hospital treatment, but includes the expense of police and court cases as well as lost working time, sickness benefits and social security payments. RoSPA has estimated that, in 1967, road accidents cost the country a total of £232 million, roughly equivalent to an average of £850 per accident. Each 1 per cent increase in accidents means a further hidden cost of over £2 million besides the tragedy, pain and anguish which is known only to those who have been involved in such situations. For these reasons alone, all road users need to become far more safety conscious.

Frequent comparisons are made with accident figures in other countries to show that our record is either better or worse, expressed in terms of casualties per 1,000 vehicles or 10,000 population. Such figures are usually meaningless, as no two countries have the same population per square mile, the same weather or the same traffic laws. In this context, Great Britain, with its population of 53 million, is usually compared with Sweden, which has a population of 8 million. That Great Britain comes off badly in such a comparison is probably owed to motorists in Sweden having more space in which to avoid hitting each other rather than to the very strict drinking laws.

Another factor which makes it very difficult to find valid

comparisons between separate countries is that deaths, serious injuries and slight injuries are classified under different rules and are not standardized. Great Britain has adopted the recommendation of the Working Party of the United Nations Economic Commission for Europe, in which the following groupings are made:

*Deaths:* people reported killed if death occurs within 30 days of the accident.

*Serious Injury:* where a person is detained as an in-patient in hospital, or has suffered from a well-defined injury requiring medical treatment.

*Slight Injury:* is an injury of a minor nature like a bruise or sprain. Shock is not included under this heading unless medical treatment has been required.

It is not yet possible to comment on long-term results from the introduction of breath tests, as this requires figures from at least three complete years before true trends can be established. In addition, there are often several months' delay before the Ministry of Transport is able to produce final figures for accidents occurring in any particular month. This means that, to date, complete figures are never possible at any time and conclusions have to be based upon either provisional figures or incomplete data.

The figures in Table 1, kindly supplied by the Royal Society for the Prevention of Accidents, show the casualty figures for the first two complete years following the introduction of breath tests. The percentage figures in brackets show the reduction, or increase, compared with the figure for the corresponding month in the year October 1966 to September 1967 before the breath test was imposed.

In the first year of the breath test (October 1967 to September 1968), the overall casualty figures showed a reduction of 14·6 per cent (1,152) deaths, 11·4 per cent (11,177) seriously injured, and 10 per cent (28,130) slightly injured. For the second year the corresponding reductions are 10·3 per cent (814) deaths, 9·0 per cent (8,841) seriously injured and 9·9 per cent (27,855) slightly injured. From these figures, it is apparent that the breath test and the 80 mg. limit are still having a definite influence upon the accident rate, but that this was not as great in the second year as in the first.

Table 1. The first two years with breath tests

| 1967 | Deaths | Seriously injured | Slightly injured |
|---|---|---|---|
| October | 594 (− 14·2%) | 7,675 (− 13·6%) | 22,726 (− 11·0%) |
| November | 639 (− 19·5%) | 7,292 (− 15·4%) | 20,949 (− 12·6%) |
| December | 654 (− 33·3%) | 7,541 (− 22·0%) | 21,512 (− 20·1%) |
| *1968* | | | |
| January | 498 (− 16·7%) | 6,251 (− 11·5%) | 17,136 (− 13·6%) |
| February | 506 (− 19·2%) | 6,119 (− 11·9%) | 18,054 (−  8·1%) |
| March | 549 (−  9·3%) | 6,930 (−  9·4%) | 20,014 (−  8·8%) |
| April | 449 (− 12·6%) | 6,572 (−  7·8%) | 19,694 (−  5·8%) |
| May | 514 (−  7·9%) | 7,192 (− 16·6%) | 21,041 (− 15·5%) |
| June | 535 (−  3·3%) | 7,519 (−  4·5%) | 22,218 (−  1·1%) |
| July | 568 (− 14·1%) | 7,957 (−  9·9%) | 22,728 (−  9·8%) |
| August | 620 (+  1·5%) | 8,222 (−  5·3%) | 23,297 (−  4·3%) |
| September | 620 (− 12·2%) | 7,966 (−  5·8%) | 22,642 (−  7·2%) |
| October | 629 (−  9·1%) | 8,086 (−  9·0%) | 22,662 (− 11·4%) |
| November | 658 (− 17·1%) | 7,952 (−  7·7%) | 22,173 (−  7·5%) |
| December | 664 (− 32·3%) | 7,797 (− 19·4%) | 22,176 (− 17·9%) |
| *1969* | | | |
| January | 611 (+  2·2%) | 7,386 (+  4·5%) | 19,561 (−  1·4%) |
| February | 443 (− 28·3%) | 6,020 (− 13·3%) | 16,929 (− 13·8%) |
| March | 504 (− 15·8%) | 6,496 (− 15·0%) | 18,004 (− 18·0%) |
| April | 521 (+  1·4%) | 6,792 (−  4·8%) | 19,011 (−  4·3%) |
| May | 559 (+  0·2%) | 7,794 (−  9·6%) | 22,652 (−  9·1%) |
| June | 539 (−  2·5%) | 7,506 (−  4·6%) | 21,219 (−  5·1%) |
| July | 667 (+  0·9%) | 7,952 (−  9·9%) | 23,034 (−  8·6%) |
| August | 623 (+  2·0%) | 8,040 (−  0·7%) | 23,358 (−  4·4%) |
| September | 666 (−  5·7%) | 7,751 (−  8·3%) | 21,507 (− 13·4%) |

Although other road safety measures undoubtedly contributed to the drop in casualties, the figures must be considered in comparison with earlier years. Between 1963 and 1966 there was an average annual increase in casualties of 4·4 per cent of deaths, 3·7 per cent of serious injuries and 2 per cent of slight injuries. The figures for the complete calendar year of 1967 are themselves exceptional, as they show a downward trend of about 4 per cent. The bulk of this decrease was owing to the inclusion of three months when the breath test was in force, but it also indicates that other road safety measures were having some effect.

It is, however, noticeable that the reduction in road casualties was little short of remarkable in the twelve months after tests were introduced. For the first few months, the casualty figures were far lower than might have been expected as people were uncertain what to expect and were particularly temperate until the nature of police action was more fully understood. Certainly there are today fewer vacant spaces in the car parks of public houses than there were in the weeks before Christmas 1967. The most recent accident figures seem, in fact, to be approaching the original reduction of 5 per cent estimated by RoSPA. As the general trend of road accidents over the years has been to increase at a fairly steady rate, it can be assumed that the true effect of the breath test has probably been even greater than appears from the casualty figures.

During the early months of 1969, claims were made that the effect of the breath test law was wearing off. Remarks of this kind tended to be based upon one month's figures taken in isolation or else implied that the 1969 figures should show a further reduction over 1968. What has been impressive is the indication that the overall accident rate remains below the level which existed before the breath test was imposed, despite the continued increase in traffic and the dark winter mornings owing to British Standard Time. If the improvement fails to be maintained, the Minister of Transport still has an option open to impose a 50 mg. level in an effort to reduce the accident figures again.

As the accident figures indicate, it would be wrong to assume that breath testing has been the only reason for the reduction of road casualties. Tyre-tread laws, safety belts, better lighting, road improvements and driver education have all contributed to safer travelling conditions, but none of the other measures have coincided with such a radical drop in the accident rate as has the introduction of breath tests.

One result of the breath test has been apparently to increase the amount of drinking within the home. As accident proneness applies under all circumstances, it would be interesting to see if there has been any corresponding increase in home accident figures as a result. But it may be that at home one is inclined to sink into an armchair after drinking, rather than indulging in some such active pursuit as running over people with a lawn mower or amputating one's fingers with a circular saw.

That alcohol does lead to accidents in quarters other than on the roads is shown by the present concern in the U.S. over aircraft accidents. It has been estimated that in at least forty-five fatal accidents involving private planes in 1968, alcohol was a major factor. The combination of even a small intake of alcohol with the decreased amount of oxygen which occurs at high altitudes leads to a pronounced impairment effect on the pilot and greatly enhances the likelihood of his making an error of judgement.

CHAPTER FOUR

# The Nature of the Breathalyser

As is explained in detail in Appendix A, ethyl alcohol can undergo several chemical reactions in which a coloured reagent is either destroyed or formed. These changes are usually carried out in solution as reactions on solid media are often difficult to apply. It would be, however, obviously undesirable for the police to have to carry solutions around with them, since spillage could easily occur once the tubes or bottles were opened. For the purpose of the screening test in Great Britain, the Ministry of Transport and the Home Office have laid down a series of basic requirements that any form of breath test apparatus must satisfy before it can be accepted for use by the police. These criteria were published in a Home Office press release in February 1967, before the 80 mg. limit came into force, so that manufacturers could submit devices for consideration.

Any acceptable apparatus must be portable, robust and small enough to be carried by police in cars or on motor-cycles. The test must be easily applied and give rapid results which are accurate enough to indicate if a suspect has a blood alcohol level 'clearly above the prescribed limit'. In addition, the apparatus must be sealed before use and not affected by any alcoholic atmosphere during storage.

These requirements from the start automatically limited the number of possible instruments quite rigorously. Many of the larger forms of apparatus used in the U.S. were immediately excluded from consideration as they could not be carried on a motor-cycle without difficulty; others were eliminated because they were more than just screening tests. Of all the many forms of detector that have been described in the scientific literature, the only one that obviously fitted the requirements and which was at the same time cheap to manufacture in large numbers was the bag and tube that has become known throughout Great Britain as the 'Breathalyser'.

This particular apparatus, currently used for all breath tests in Great Britain, is manufactured under the registered trade mark 'Alcotest 80' and is based upon a colour change reaction involving a potassium dichromate/sulphuric acid mixture. The difficulties of carrying around solutions of chemical reagents for breath tests were appreciated in the early 1950s in Germany, where a simple device was required for roadside screening purposes. Research on different procedures led the Drägerwerk Company in Lübeck, who are specialists in methods of detecting small quantities of gases and vapours, to manufacture an apparatus in which the reagents are impregnated on a solid support and retained in a sealed glass tube. Many difficulties exist in producing the chemicals in a form which will give a consistently sensitive and accurate reaction. As a result, several patents exist in different countries which detail modifications to the elementary system and which claim to give greater sensitivity or more distinctive colour changes. This particular apparatus was used in Germany for more than fifteen years, and also in Sweden and Austria, before being adopted in Great Britain in 1967.

Typical of the constitution of breath tubes is that listed in the U.S. patent granted to K. Grosskopf in 1960. In this, the inert solid support is specified as being silica gel. Sulphuric acid and potassium dichromate are mixed with the silica gel and a small quantity of both arsenious oxide and iodine are added to the mixture. Before it can be packed into tubes, the impregnated solid is heated at $100-200°C$. to give a granular solid material that is yellow-orange in colour.

As the Home Office requires that the chemicals must be in a sealed container before use, no breathalyser employed by the police should be opened until directly before being used as exposure to the atmosphere can lead to a partial colour change occurring and an erroneously high reading of breath alcohol being obtained. The complete breathalyser kit before use is shown in Figure 2.

The mouthpiece (A) is of plastic and is kept in a sealed container before being used. It is designed to give a close fit when pushed on to the glass tube (B). The chemically impregnated silica gel is held in place in the tube, which measures about three inches (8 cm.) in length and three-eighths of an inch (1 cm.) in diameter, by means of pieces of fine wire mesh. To ensure that the tube is used the correct way round, it is marked with an arrow to show the direction in which the air

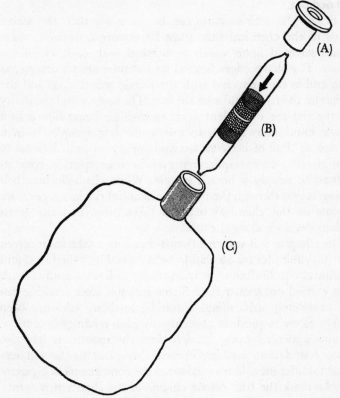

Figure 2. The breathalyser kit

should be blown and has a white band at the blowing end and a yellow band at the bag end. Another yellow line marked around the circumference of the tube about half-way along the length of the silica gel indicates the 80 mg. limit. If the breath alcohol leads to a colour change beyond this mark, then the test is considered positive and the motorist is likely to be taken to the police station for further testing. The third part of the apparatus, the plastic bag (c), is connected to a short piece of rubber tubing to form a closely fitting seal with the lower end of the glass tube. It is usual for one bag to be used for about ten tests before being replaced. This extended usage should give rise to no errors so long as the bag is properly flattened out before the apparatus is assembled, and the test carried out.

Before the various parts can be fitted together, the sealed ends of the chemical tube must be removed, usually with a small serrated knife which is supplied with each kit of ten tubes. The sharp edges formed on the tube are no danger, as one end is then covered with the plastic mouthpiece and the other by the rubber tube on the bag. The success and reliability of the test are dependent upon enough air being blown in a single continuous breath to inflate the bag completely in a period of time of between ten and twenty seconds. Refusal to comply with these requirements has been accepted in court as refusal to supply a breath sample. While alcoholic breath is being blown through the tube, a substantial rise in temperature occurs as the chemical reaction takes place and the green colour develops along the tube.

In Chapter 2 it was mentioned that it can take from fifteen to thirty minutes for alcohol to be absorbed into the blood and a state of equilibrium to be reached. For this reason, any breath test carried out sooner than fifteen minutes after drinking can be completely misleading. Similarly, anybody who has been sick is likely to produce anomalously high readings because of stomach alcohol being brought into the mouth. It has also been found that smoking immediately prior to the test can lead to different colour reactions as the constituents of cigarette smoke mask the true colour change of the chemical reagents. Such methods of confusing the test as sucking peppermints or drinking water or coffee are of no value since they have been shown to have no effect upon the alcohol already absorbed into the blood stream.

It has been established that simply eating or drinking large quantities of fruit or fruit juices can lead to a slightly higher than normal blood alcohol figure. However, nobody existing on a diet of fruit and juices is likely to give a positive breath test, as it takes at least a pound of fruit to raise the blood alcohol level by as little as 8 mg./100 ml., and it would be necessary to consume about eleven pounds of fruit in one hour to risk reaching the limit. The breath test is not concerned with the origin of the alcohol it detects, and, as far as the inability to drive matters, alcohol from one source is as dangerous as alcohol from another.

Our current breath-testing device can be manufactured to give a measurable response to levels of alcohol as low as 30 mg./100 ml., and will in fact give a colour change with a level of 5 mg./100 ml. Any alteration of the legal limit in this country would simply necessitate shifting the position of the yellow line on the tube and not changing to a different form of screening test.

Considerable conflict exists over the level of accuracy that can be expected from the 'Alcotest 80'. The advocates of the method claim that the green zone produced increases roughly in the same proportion as the breath alcohol (and hence the blood alcohol) concentration. In support of this contention, Dr Grosskopf has shown that 98 per cent of test subjects with more than 80 mg./100 ml. gave a positive result on the 'Alcotest 80'. His results also showed that 5 per cent of test subjects with blood alcohol levels around 50 mg./100 ml. gave a positive result. Only when the blood alcohol level was below 50 mg./100 ml., did the test subjects give all results below the 80 mg. mark on the tube.

Within the first month of its application in Great Britain, of the 927 drivers who gave a positive reaction at the kerbside, 168 (18 per cent) were below the 80 mg. level on analysis of the blood or urine samples. While some of these may have fallen below the limit during the delays before testing, it appears that the possible error on the breath tube is quite high. Research carried out by Dr G. G. Muir and his colleagues supports this contention. Their work, published in *Nature* on 6 September 1968, showed that 77 per cent of their subjects giving positive breath tests using the 'Alcotest 80' apparatus actually had blood alcohol levels below the 80 mg. limit. Even more serious was the observation that 62 per cent of the subjects possessing less than 50 mg./100 ml. failed the breath test. Results such as these have given rise to considerable comment in the national press, and it is obvious that people in general are becoming less and less satisfied with the results of breath tests as they are currently carried out.

Although the Home Office has emphasized that the breath test is only a preliminary step, its value even as a screening device is open to question when errors as great as those quoted are observed. Various figures which have been produced in Parliament show that the Home Office is aware that between 16 to 24 per cent of breath tests are giving positive results when blood alcohol levels are below the prescribed limit.

Although the roadside breath test does not have to be one hundred per cent accurate, it is essential that any degree of error should be kept to a minimum and act to the advantage of the motorist rather than against him. Any test which gives incorrectly high readings will lead to a large number of motorists being asked to go to the police station to give blood or urine samples which, on analysis, will show results below the limit. The wasted time and effort involved in this could be considerable.

The extent of the colour change in the breath tube depends upon two things: first, the amount of alcohol in the breath, and secondly, the amount of breath blown through the tube. As the first of these represents the object being investigated, it is necessary that the second should be a firmly established volume. In theory, this is achieved by the plastic bag being blown to its fullest extent, that is, to a constant fixed volume. It is, therefore, apparent that any variation in bag sizes can produce misleading results. So far there is no indication that any investigations on the accuracy of the tests have taken this potential source of error into consideration.

Two particular modified forms of the standard type of breath tube have been patented in Great Britain. The first, by T. Kitagawa (British patent 1,011,929), uses tubes five inches (12 cm.) in length and one fifteenth of an inch (1·8 mm.) in diameter which contain chromium trioxide and sulphuric acid on silica particles. The chemical reaction in the tube is essentially the same as that used at present, giving a colour change from yellow to blue. Owing to the thinner, longer tube and changed inert support, it is claimed that no error is greater than 10 per cent. For a screening device, this is considered very good and is an apparent improvement upon the 'Alcotest 80'. Unfortunately, the modification has the disadvantage that it must be used at an elevated temperature of about 50°C.

(122°F.), which limits its potential use to incorporation in a less portable system incorporating a heating unit.

The other modification, by D. Julita and J. Hayoz (British patent 1,070,199), uses a flattened tube in which suitable reagents are impregnated on a strip of cardboard or plastic. Any reaction with alcohol when breath is blown through the tube takes place on the strip's surface. For this system the advantage is claimed that it is easier to read the colour change accurately because of the larger surface area.

The general public should be cautious about purchasing any of the numerous imitations of the 'Alcotest 80' which have flooded the market. Many of these are poorly made and highly inaccurate. In some cases they may lead a person to believe he is fit to drive when in fact he is not. Unless the device states the level of accuracy which can be expected and the other factors that can affect the result, it is not worth the expense. In at least one case magistrates found a driver guilty although he had driven only because his self-applied breath test had indicated that he was below the limit.

CHAPTER FIVE

# Other Forms of Breath-Testing Apparatus

Many varied forms of breath-testing apparatus have been made and patented in different countries around the world. For the most part, they are far more cumbersome than that currently used in Great Britain. The U.S. has been the home of the major developments in this field, mainly because each of the fifty states is individually responsible for establishing its drinking and driving laws and the form of breath test apparatus, if any, that is used to implement those laws. In many cases, the apparatuses described in this chapter are used for quantitative, conclusive tests rather than for screening purposes, and results from them are frequently employed directly as evidence of driving under the influence in the countries where they are used. In this case an apparatus will tend to be more precise and more highly refined and sophisticated than the simple breath tube.

*The Intoximeter*, shown diagrammatically in Figure 3, was originally developed in the U.S. in 1941 (U.S. patent 2,591,691) and has been used extensively as an on-the-spot test for blood alcohol levels.

This apparatus consists of a balloon (A) connected by a divided tube (B) to a glass section in which a solution of acidified potassium permanganate is retained in a sintered glass portion of the tube, and to a second branch consisting of a pre-weighed tube of magnesium perchlorate (C) joined in series with a similar tube (D) containing Ascarite (sodium hydroxide on shredded asbestos).

The balloon is inflated by continuous blowing, and when full the mouthpiece is stoppered. The plug at the end of the tube (B) is removed and air from the balloon allowed to pass slowly through the oxidizing reagents for a set period of time. The quantity of potassium permanganate reagent is calculated in such a way that, if the alcohol in the expired breath is above a predefined level, the purple colour of the chemicals is completely removed during the time in which the breath is allowed to pass through. The remainder of the expired breath

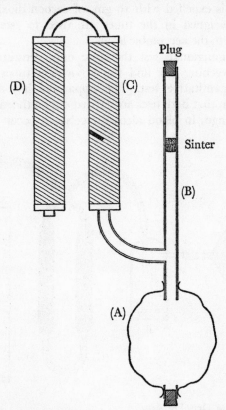

Figure 3. The Intoximeter

in the balloon is then passed through the magnesium perchlorate tube (c) in which the alcohol and water vapour are absorbed, and then through the Ascarite tube (D), where the carbon dioxide reacts with the sodium hydroxide.

If the breath sample has totally removed the colour of the potassium permanganate, the whole apparatus is sent to a laboratory for further study to be made on the absorbed substances. The quantity of alcohol absorbed by the magnesium perchlorate is determined by chemical analysis and is related to the weight of carbon dioxide absorbed in the Ascarite. On the basis of the equilibrium which exists between alcohol in the breath and alcohol in the blood, it has been determined that the amount of alcohol present in 100 ml. of blood is equal to that which is expelled with 19 gm. of carbon dioxide. So the quantities weighed in the tubes are used to establish their relationship to the acceptable levels.

The permanganate test therefore only constitutes a preliminary screening test and the absorption tubes the more accurate quantitative test. The apparatus has an obvious advantage in that both tests are carried out on the same sample and no changes in blood alcohol levels can occur because of delay.

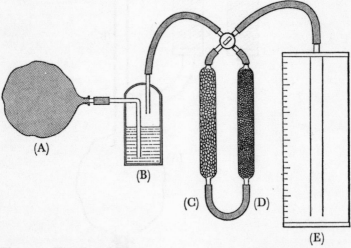

Figure 4. The Drunkometer

*The Drunkometer* is another device invented and patented in the U.S. (U.S. patent 2,867,511). It is a rather elaborate balloon and pump design in which exhaled breath is first collected, then pumped through a mixed solution of potassium permanganate and sulphuric acid, as shown diagrammatically in Figure 4.

The balloon (A), initially detached from the main apparatus, is blown up with expired air. When full, it is attached to the tube leading to the reagent solution (B). The chemical concentration of the solution is chosen so that it will be decolourized by reaction with a predefined amount of alcohol. A sample of breath from the balloon is passed through the acidified potassium permanganate until the solution is virtually colourless. After passing through the solution, the air is carried through the drying tube (c) and then through the Ascarite tube (D) in which the expired carbon dioxide is absorbed. Finally, the volume of air is measured by means of a water-filled gasometer (E).

The amount of alcohol known to decolourize the reagent solution can be directly related to the volume of breath measured by the gasometer, and hence by direct relationship to the blood alcohol content. Alternatively, the blood alcohol content can be calculated from the amount of carbon dioxide absorbed in the Ascarite tube, on the same basis as for the Intoximeter (page 33).

This particular apparatus has been used both for screening and for quantitative testing. It includes controls which enable sections not required to be isolated from the main body of the device.

*The Alcometer*, first described and manufactured in the U.S. in 1941, is based upon the pumping of a measured sample of breath through a heated tube which contains iodine pentoxide. Oxidation of the alcohol leads to the release of iodine vapour, which is then passed into a solution of starch and potassium iodide. The quantity of iodine formed during the oxidation depends upon the amount of alcohol present, and this leads to a blue coloration in the starch/potassium iodine solution that relates to the original concentration of alcohol. The apparatus is designed to give an automatic reading of the intensity of the blue colour, and the amount of alcohol to which this corresponds is read off from a calibrated dial.

In the simplified diagram (Figure 5), air is blown through the mouthpiece (A) and retained in the tube (B). After adjusting the control valves, the complete measured sample is then pumped, by means of purified air, through the hot iodine pentoxide tube (c), any iodine released being automatically carried into the starch/potassium iodine solution (D). The tube in which the colour reaction takes place is fitted into an optical system (E) between a lamp and photoelectric cell that responds to the blue intensity of the solution and converts the reading on the meter to the amount of alcohol that has brought about the reaction.

This apparatus suffers from the disadvantage of it being necessary to heat the iodine pentoxide tube, which may take several minutes starting from cold. A complete analysis for quantitative purposes by this method may take nearly twenty minutes.

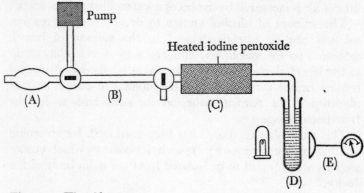

Figure 5. The Alcometer

*The Breathalyzer.* It is unfortunate that this name, although spelt differently, has become the colloquial term for the device currently employed in Great Britain. The apparatus to which it correctly refers was originally described in 1957 and is covered by British patent no. 821,013 granted in 1959. The apparatus, shown diagrammatically in Figure 6, has been used extensively in the United States, Canada and Australia both for screening and for conclusive quantitative results to be used in court.

Breath is blown into the apparatus, thus causing the piston (A) to rise to the top of the cylinder (B). By altering the control valve (c), the measured volume is then forced, by the falling piston, through a heated solution of potassium dichromate and sulphuric acid (D). Any alcohol present in the breath causes the formation of green chromium sulphate. The intensity of the colour change is related to the amount of alcohol in the breath and is compared to a standard (E), the absolute value being measured on the photoelectric circuit. The meter (F) is calibrated to give a direct reading of the concentration of alcohol in the blood on the basis of its relationship to the breath alcohol content. An aluminium case houses the apparatus, which incorporates a heating unit to warm the breath sample to 50°C. (122°F.) and the test ampoules to 65°C. (149°F.) before any analysis is carried out.

The advocates of this particular apparatus claim a level of accuracy for it which compares with direct blood alcohol analytical figures.

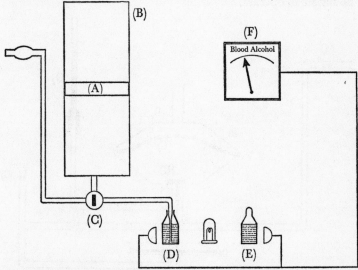

Figure 6. The Breathalyzer

*Wright–Kitagawa Apparatus.* In 1962 B. M. Wright and T. Kitagawa criticized all the systems in which corrosive chemical solutions were used on the grounds of the difficulties which arise in disposing of the waste tubes. Together they devised an apparatus to incorporate the tubes of chromic acid deposited upon silica particles patented by Professor Kitagawa (page 30). The tube, contained in a box that can be heated to 60°C. (140°F.), gives a colour change along its length that increases with any increase in breath alcohol. A linear relationship between the length of the colour change and alcohol content exists for levels between 50 and 200 mg./100 ml. blood. In the apparatus, shown in simplified form in Figure 7, breath blown through tube A is arranged to by-pass the reservoir (B). Owing to the constriction (C), a slight build-up of pressure occurs and causes the diaphragm (D) to rise and lift the valve (E). Breath then enters the reservoir, moving the diaphragm (F) to give a fixed volume of 100 ml. which is forced through the reagent tube (G). Various controls and valves are built into the apparatus to ensure that the breath passes through the appropriate section at the correct time.

This apparatus has already been used in an exploratory manner in several British police stations and has been shown to be simple to operate.

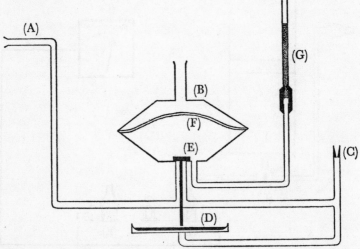

Figure 7. Wright–Kitagawa Apparatus

*Gas-Liquid Chromatography Apparatus.* One of the most sensitive methods of analysis, known as gas-liquid chromatography (G.L.C.), is described in detail in Chapter 7, but this rather cumbersome laboratory procedure has also been ingeniously adapted to give a portable form for use as an on-the-spot testing device (U.S. patent 3,338,087). For this purpose, the driver's breath is collected by blowing into a large specially calibrated syringe from which a measured volume is pumped to be studied by the G.L.C. method. The various gaseous constituents of the breath, including the alcohol, are detected by a process known as thermal conductivity, in which the temperature and electrical resistance of a hot wire are varied depending upon the nature of the gas passing over it. The disadvantages of the method are that it needs both a supply of an unreactive gas, such as helium, and a constant source of electricity.

\*

All quantitative methods of detection suffer from limitations and have varying degrees of accuracy, and a statistical study can easily establish the accuracy that is to be expected from any particular method. Any person, be he judge, jury or scientist, who has reason to refer to such results, should ensure that he is informed on the accuracy to be expected as well as the absolute value obtained.

To take one example, an investigation into the accuracy of the Wright–Kitagawa apparatus against that for the Breathalyzer (U.S.), carried out in 1964, showed the former to be accurate to within $\pm 8 \cdot 5$ mg./100 ml., as against $\pm 7$ mg./ 100 ml. for the latter. Neither of these methods was as accurate as values obtained by laboratory analysis of the corresponding blood samples where the limitation was $\pm 3 \cdot 5$ mg./100 ml.

As the Home Office has not specifically excluded more elaborate devices than the one currently employed, it is very likely that eventually the breath tube will be displaced from its pre-eminent position by an instrument similar to one of those described above. Before such instruments are likely to be accepted for anything other than preliminary screening tests in Great Britain, however, their levels of accuracy and reproducibility will need to be greatly improved. As things stand, the simple breath tube currently employed is likely to take a lot of beating on the grounds of economy and convenience.

# CHAPTER SIX

# Samples at the Police Station

The delay in reaching an equilibrium of alcohol distribution in body tissue, mentioned in Chapter 2, does not in itself invalidate the sampling of breath, blood and urine. For a reasonably accurate on-the-spot test, a breath sample is the obvious choice as the expired air is in a constant state of equilibrium from the blood passing through the lungs. As blood or urine samples are taken under medical supervision only after fairly lengthy delays at the police station, conditions of equilibrium are almost certainly reached in all cases. Any delays in sampling are likely to act to the advantage of the driver, who steadily uses up the alcohol in his system all the time.

In many cases, where a sample is required for analysis, the person under investigation frequently chooses to supply urine in preference to blood, even though the law requires that he be asked for a blood sample first. This preference is mainly because of the greater ease of supplying an adequate sample rather than because it is likely to produce a more accurate figure. In actual fact, however, all the evidence suggests that urine is less capable of giving reliable figures than blood.

The errors that can occur with urine samples arise partially from the time-lapse in alcohol being eliminated from the body fluids into the bladder, and partially from variations in observed values for converting urine alcohol figures to blood alcohol figures.

The legal limit for alcohol in urine, as specified by the Road Safety Act of 1967, is 107 mg./100 ml., and this is considered to be equivalent to a blood alcohol level of 80 mg./100 ml. on the basis of a 1·33 conversion factor. The origin and justification of this particular value has come under strong criticism on several occasions. As long ago as 1948, it was shown that the conversion factor could vary between 1·2 and 1·4, depending upon the specific gravity* of the urine. A statistical survey of 10,000 blood and urine test cases, carried out in 1962 by Dr W. Froentjes, showed that there was a very poor correlation on the 1·33 urine/blood conversion factor and that a more correct figure would be of the order of 1·52 or higher. During 1967, the report of a similar comparative study was published in the *British Medical Journal* by Professor J. P. Payne and colleagues. This showed that there is virtually no simple correlation between the figures for alcohol in urine and those for alcohol in blood sampled at the same time. The factors varied from about 1·00 to 2·50, and averaged out to 1·44: still higher than the accepted 1·33. These research workers consider that the use of the urine to blood alcohol conversion ratio of 1·33:1 is unjustified as the analysis of urine cannot give an accurate assessment of the blood alcohol level.

The consensus of specialized opinion in this field of work is strongly against the use of urine samples for estimating blood alcohol levels. As the central nervous system is affected by the alcohol in the blood and not by that in the urine, the law should primarily be concerned with the former. It is quite obvious that, under the present system, it is possible for a person to be convicted with more than the prescribed limit of alcohol in his urine when it could be that he would be below the limit on a corresponding blood sample. A clear case seems to exist to justify further studies on the relationship between blood and urine alcohol levels before the 1·33 figure is accepted as absolute. It has also been suggested that the taking of urine samples for the purpose of establishing alcohol levels should be discontinued, and that only results obtained from blood samples, taken under rigorous conditions, should be admissible as evidence in court.

At present, samples of blood are taken in one of two possible ways; either as capillary blood, by squeezing out a few drops from a pin-prick in an ear lobe or thumb, or by syringe from a vein. These methods were the subject of a penetrating article by Graham Chedd in the *New Scientist* in March 1968. The

* Specific gravity is defined as the weight of a known volume of a substance compared to the weight of the same volume of water.

article referred extensively to Professor Payne's work, criticizing the sampling procedures and casting doubt upon the reliability of pin-prick samples.

Criticism is based upon four possible sources of error:

(a) Capillary blood is likely to give a high alcohol value, as it contains proportionally more plasma than does venous blood.
(b) While the drops are being squeezed from the finger, alcohol is likely to evaporate, thus leading to a lower figure.
(c) As the sample containers are only partially filled, evaporation continues from the surface of the sample into the void volume above until such a time as the sample is refrigerated. This, again, contributes to a lower alcohol figure.
(d) Some samples clot inside the containers despite the presence of anti-coagulants, and any test therefore tends to be carried out on the plasma-enriched fluid portion and so gives rise to a higher alcohol figure.

To eliminate these possible sources of error, it would be necessary to take more adequate precautions with sampling in general. Specimens of blood should only be taken from veins, by means of a hypodermic syringe, and the sample tubes containing excess anti-coagulant should be completely filled before being fitted with their air-tight cap. Despite these criticisms, the practice of taking pin-prick samples has continued, and in November 1969 the (then new) Minister of Transport, Mr F. Mulley, was photographed giving a blood sample by this procedure.

Even the preparation for sampling by means of a hypodermic syringe is open to errors which must be carefully guarded against. In any application of needle to skin, it is normal to disinfect the surface beforehand with aqueous alcohol. When the object of the sampling is to investigate the alcoholic content of the blood, it is obvious that disinfection by this method can justifiably lead to a contention that a high blood alcohol level results from the skin's absorption of the disinfecting fluid. This possible source of error has been recognized for many years and various studies made of it. For similar reasons, ether, iodine and phenolic solutions cannot be employed. Because of this, the recommended disinfectant for blood sampling is a 1 per cent solution of mercuric chloride; this provides adequate protection without carrying a risk of producing misleading results.

It will be apparent that obtaining an accurate sample of blood for laboratory testing can be a very involved process, and the difficulties go a long way to explain the preference for urine which sometimes exists. When it is remembered that, at the least, a person's pleasure, or even his livelihood, can depend upon the result of a test for alcohol, it is essential that every effort should be made to achieve the utmost accuracy. If any reliability is to be placed upon results of samples, it is necessary that the many potential sources of error be eliminated. The value of scientific methods to the community depends upon their correct application; the evidence available suggests very strongly that, at the present time, drivers are being convicted on evidence which derives from what can only be called a cheap imitation of scientific investigation.

# CHAPTER SEVEN

# The Testing of Samples

When a sample, whether of urine or blood, has been taken, it proceeds along a fairly well-established route. To prevent deterioration, it is refrigerated at the earliest opportunity and kept in this condition until immediately before analysis.

The amount of alcohol in the sample may be determined by one of three main methods:

(a) Chemical procedures in which any alcohol present is converted into other compounds and the quantities established by means of a colour-change reaction.
(b) Chemico-physical methods in which alcohol is separated from other components of the sample and the amounts of each assessed from measurements on a chart record sheet.
(c) Biochemical methods in which the alcohol is digested by means of an enzymatic reaction.

Methods employed for chemical analysis have been carefully developed over many years, most approaches being established long before the law was concerned with this particular application of science. The recommended procedures adopted for the study of alcohol in body fluids were laid down by a committee formed by the British Medical Association in conjunction with the Royal Institute of Chemistry. This committee, under the chairmanship of Dr D. W. Kent-Jones, produced its report in 1954 and recommended two chemical analytical procedures for use by trained analysts for the general investigation of alcohol in body fluids.

These two main methods, named after the scientists responsible for most of the development work, are:

(a) The Cavett micro-method, employing only 0·1 ml. of urine or blood for the complete analysis.
(b) The Kozelka and Hine macro-method in which a 1–2 ml. sample is necessary.

The first uses a specially made flask about 8 cm. (3 in.) high and with a 5 cm. (2 in.) diameter base, as shown in Figure 8.

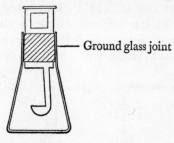

Ground glass joint

Figure 8. The Cavett micro-method analysis apparatus

Carefully measured quantities of potassium dichromate solution and concentrated sulphuric acid are placed in the flask. The urine or blood sample is measured into the small glass cup suspended from the flask's ground-glass stopper. After careful sealing, the contents of the flask are gently heated at 37°C. (99°F.) for about four hours, during which time the oxidation of the alcohol in the sample uses up a certain amount of the potassium dichromate. By determining the quantity of potassium dichromate remaining at the end of the four hours, it is possible to calculate the amount used and hence the amount of alcohol in the sample.

Determinations of this type are never carried out in isolation; two or more consistent results are necessary before an analyst can be satisfied that the result is accurate.

Although the Kozelka and Hine method also involves oxidation of alcohol, it differs in two major respects from the Cavett method: (a) it involves a sample ten to twenty times as large; and (b) the alcohol is separated from the other constituents of the sample before being chemically treated. The procedure requires that the sample, contained in the long glass tube shown on the left-hand side in Figure 9, is heated on a hot-water bath with steam being simultaneously passed through it from a steam generator. Thus the alcohol is steam distilled through the apparatus to the second tube and eventually to the condenser, where the aqueous solution is condensed and collected.

A total volume of about 25 ml. of water and alcohol is collected from the distillation apparatus and accurately measured quantities of potassium dichromate and sulphuric acid are added to the flask. After being sealed, the flask is heated at 100°C. (212°F.) for twenty minutes. The amount of alcohol in the original sample is then calculated from the quantity of potassium dichromate which has been used up in the chemical reaction in a similar way to the Cavett method.

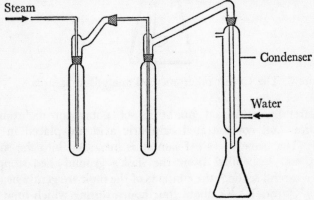

Figure 9. The Kozelka and Hine steam-distillation apparatus

The committee responsible for recommending these two methods emphasized that accuracy and reproducibility were only possible if determinations were carried out by experienced analysts employing carefully cleaned apparatus and accurately standardized chemical solutions.

It will be appreciated, even by readers who have no special knowledge of chemistry, that these methods of analysis will give incorrect results if other compounds exist in the urine or blood samples which are also capable of reacting with the potassium dichromate/sulphuric acid mixture. Fortunately, the number of possible interfering substances is very limited. Those which can interfere are a more serious problem in the Cavett method than in the Kozelka and Hine one. In the former it is necessary for the analyst to confirm the absence of such things as acetone and salicylic acid before any analysis can be carried out. In the latter, this preliminary work is not required, but blood samples must be treated with sodium tungstate solution to precipitate protein before steam distillation is carried out.

Like all analytical methods, the full value of the results depends upon a knowledge of the degree of accuracy to be expected. Obviously a result obtained by a method that is likely to be as much as, say, 20 per cent inaccurate is far less acceptable than a result obtained by a method which involves only a 5 per cent possible error.

A careful statistical analysis obtained with the two recommended methods in several different analytical laboratories was used to determine the possible levels of error. This showed that the Cavett method, carried out in duplicate, is capable of giving results which are accurate within ±10 per cent. Hence a sample giving a value of 80 mg./100 ml. on analysis could actually be as low as 72 mg. or as high as 88 mg. In a marginal case such as this, the analyst should carry out further determinations on the same sample to improve the precision of the results. The final result should, in any case, always be presented in a form that shows the level of accuracy to be expected from the figures obtained.

Similarly, the Kozelka and Hine method gave results that were accurate within ±5 per cent. In this case, a value of 80 mg. could mean a possible true value between 76 mg. and 84 mg.

It is unlikely that the levels of accuracy in these two chemical methods of analysis can be improved to any great extent. It is therefore only fair to an accused motorist that analytical results from his sample should always refer specifically to the minimum possible level of alcohol indicated within the limits of the method of analysis.

Because of these limitations on accuracy, it is possible for two analysts to obtain what are apparently entirely different results from the same sample. This has occurred in several court cases where the analyst for the defence has obtained a value lower than that obtained by the analyst for the prosecution. That this has happened should surprise nobody, but it is essential for any magistrate to be told whether these results show any relation to each other, allowing for possible errors in analysis. Without this knowledge, it is possible for a wrong emphasis to be placed on one or the other of the results and for a miscarriage of justice to occur.

It is at least reassuring to know that the number of cases involving conflicting analytical results is very small and can only constitute a minute proportion of the total number of those concerned with driving with more than the prescribed level of alcohol. Possibly, however, this is also because many motorists fail to avail themselves of the opportunity of having an independent analysis made on their sample. If this is so, it indicates either a high level of short-sightedness or public ignorance; the very techniques which exist to detect the law-breaker are also there to protect the innocent. The law has no monopoly over the scientific procedures that can be used.

The chemical methods already described for analysing samples are not the only techniques available. During the past fifteen years, research chemists have developed a highly sensitive method for separating different volatile chemicals from each other. This is the process used also for such things as detecting minute quantities of pesticides in animal tissues, known as gas-liquid chromatography (G.L.C.). Since it is sensitive to minute quantities of chemicals, the procedure can also be applied to determining amounts of alcohol in samples of blood and urine. Many analysts now use this method in preference to the rather more laborious chemical techniques. It has the added advantage that it requires far less time to train a person to use than does teaching him to obtain accurate results from the chemical methods.

Gas-liquid chromatography is really a sort of obstacle course for molecules based upon the various physical and chemical properties of substances in a sample. In its simplest form, the apparatus consists of a glass tube about two to three feet long packed with a granular material that might be anything from powdered brick to chalk. The powder is used as a support medium for a thick, viscous, non-volatile liquid such as a silicone oil. A continuous flow of gas, usually a mixture of hydrogen and helium or nitrogen, is passed through the column from one end to the other, the rate of flow being carefully regulated by flow meters.

To analyse volatile mixtures, only minute quantities of the order of 1–2 microlitres (a millionth part of a litre) are required. Measurement of these small amounts in a sample is achieved by a specially constructed syringe, and the exact quantity is injected into the gas flow immediately before it enters the column. By this means, the mixture is carried through the column. Owing to the physical and chemical differences that exist between species of molecules, they move along the column at different rates, and what was originally a mixture is separated into its molecular components. As the hydrogen and helium or nitrogen carrier gas leaves the column, it passes through a detector system in which the hydrogen and sample components are burnt and identified by electrical conductivity. This detector gives a constant reading when only pure carrier gas is passing through it, but whenever one of the components of the mixture is carried out of the column the reading changes. The detector is linked to a pen recorder, which automatically shows the appearance of individual components as a series of peaks traced on a moving roll of chart paper. The sizes of the peaks on the chart are proportional to the relative amounts of each component in the original mixture.

If the G.L.C. column is operated with an established gas flow, under carefully controlled conditions, a particular chemical compound will always take the same time to pass through it. This time, referred to as the 'retention time', is used as the basis for identifying compounds in various mixtures. In practice, the retention times for chemical compounds are established by using pure materials, which then set a standard for identifying the same components in mixtures. As the peak area is directly related to the amount of the compound applied to the column, it therefore becomes possible to establish the amount of any volatile substance in a solution, and this remains the case with alcohol in blood and urine.

The flow diagram (Figure 10) indicates the arrangement of a G.L.C. apparatus and shows the type of chart record obtained.

Several techniques have been used to apply samples to the head of the G.L.C. column. As urine samples are almost completely volatile, it is possible to inject them directly on to the head of the column. In the case of blood, however, directly injecting the sample can, after a time, lead to a blockage of the injection unit owing to an accumulation of non-volatile residues. Because of this, the alcohol in blood samples is often transferred to a more suitable medium, either by extraction with another solvent, such as butanol, or by exchange with a measured quantity of air, before being injected.

To improve the accuracy of the G.L.C. technique, it is usual for analysts to add a measured amount of another chemical (such as acetone or acetaldehyde) to the sample under examination. By this means, the amount of alcohol can, by the size of its chart peak, be related to the corresponding peak size which is obtained from the known amount of the internal standard.

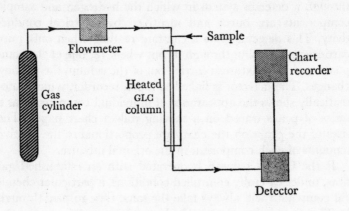

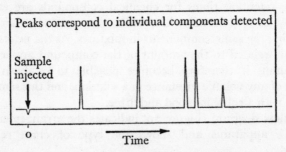

Figure 10. (*Top*) A flow diagram for the technique of gas-liquid chromatography, with (*below*) a typical chart record

Typical column conditions for determining alcohol samples employ helium gas flowing at 75 ml./minute through a 2 m. (6 ft.) column of 6 mm. ($\frac{1}{4}$ in.) diameter containing polyoxyethylene on a solid support maintained at 300°C. (572°F.). By this means, the analyst takes about thirty minutes to make a complete determination, compared with one to five hours with the chemical methods.

G.L.C. is a very sensitive method of analysis which can detect many different compounds in extremely minute quantities. Its degree of accuracy varies a great deal according to the quality of the column and the ability of the operator. The author has found, from his own lecturing and teaching experience, that it is possible to train an undergraduate student to obtain reproducible results within the acceptable limits of accuracy by two or three hours of practical instruction.

A comparison of several scientific reports shows that, in general, the range of error in gas-liquid chromatographic analysis is no greater than $\pm 5$ per cent; as good as the Kozelka and Hine chemical method and much more rapid. By the use of internal standards it is possible to improve the accuracy to $\pm 2$ per cent. Any analyst carrying out determinations will invariably carefully check his equipment for accuracy and reproducibility before studying any forensic samples, but even so the results obtained should be expressed in a way that shows the limits within which the values lie.

The biochemical method of analysis for ethyl alcohol is based upon the conversion of alcohol to acetaldehyde through the action of an organic catalyst (an enzyme), known as alcohol dehydrogenase (ADH). The method is of value because it is specific for ethyl alcohol when applied to blood or urine samples. Unfortunately, a single analysis can take between one and two hours to perform. Although an automatic procedure for the analysis of a large number of samples has been developed, the technique has not been widely adopted in this country, probably because of the pre-eminence of gas-liquid chromatography.

To help the motorist who needs an independent analysis of the sample which he retains after police examination, the Royal Institute of Chemistry has published a list of qualified analytical chemists equipped to undertake analysis of blood or urine samples. The recommended fee for this service is five guineas. Analysts who use the G.L.C. method as against the chemical methods are specially indicated on the list. For the benefit of readers, this list, correct to November 1969, is reproduced by permission of the Royal Institute of Chemistry as Appendix B.

# CHAPTER EIGHT

# Drinking, Driving and the Law

Like nearly all Acts of Parliament, the Road Safety Act 1967, including the section dealing with breath tests, is filled with turgid prose involving numerous cross-references to sub-sections of sub-sections. It is no surprise that people have been able to find loopholes through which they could crawl. The attempts of civil servants to produce a water-tight legal document from medical and scientific data have resulted in a law that looks good on paper but which has been found to be loose and vague in practice. It has been claimed that at least fifty technical loopholes exist in the breath test law. The Road Safety Act 1967 is really an extension to the Road Traffic Act 1960, and, with other related modifications, these are known collectively as the Road Traffic Acts 1960 to 1967.

In outline, the 1967 Act makes it an offence to drive or to be in charge of a motor vehicle with a blood alcohol level above 80 mg./100 ml., or a urine alcohol level of 107 mg./100 ml. For driving or attempting to drive under these conditions the penalties on conviction are: automatic disqualification from driving for one year and a possible fine of up to £100 or up to four months' imprisonment. For a subsequent conviction, the possible term of imprisonment is increased to six months and disqualification to three years.

The following are examples of cases in which drivers were successfully charged with driving with more than the prescribed amount of alcohol in their blood. In these instances the law was interpreted in the manner intended, no attempts being made to escape through technicalities:

Mr A., stopped for speeding, failed the breath test. His blood gave a reading above 170 mg. on being tested several hours

after he had drunk about four pints of beer. He was fined
£20 and disqualified for one year.

Mr B. had been drinking a mixture of beer and brandy over a
period of three hours. He failed the breath test after being
stopped for speeding. Analysis of the blood sample gave a
reading above 140 mg. When found guilty of driving with
more than the prescribed amount of alcohol, he was fined
£75.

Mr C. drank a large amount of brandy over a period of about
six hours; when tested after skidding and hitting a road sign,
his blood alcohol level was found to be over 190 mg. His
fine was £100.

Mrs D. was involved in a slight accident after having been
drinking vodka. After failing a breath test, analysis of her
blood gave a figure of 120 mg. alcohol/100 ml. She was
fined £25 and disqualified from driving for one year.

There is one point that emerges from these cases, and that is
that while the disqualification is automatic, there is no con-
sistency over the extent of the fine, the heaviness of which
varies greatly between one court and another. As this is the
only regular form of discretion open to the courts, it would
appear that such factors as previous driving records and circumstances in which alcohol has been drunk are taken into
account at this stage. Many critics of the law consider that
automatic disqualification for what may often be a first motoring offence is too severe. The alternative of a fixed fine of at
least £50, coupled with disqualification at the discretion of the
court, has often been suggested, but it is fairly certain that
under these conditions the 80 mg. limit would cease to be as
great a deterrent as it now is. Whatever else changes, it is unlikely that the penalties will be eased.

Automatic disqualification already exists under the Road
Traffic Act 1962 for a variety of offences, including causing
death by dangerous driving and also for dangerous driving
within three years of a previous conviction for dangerous driving or for driving while disqualified. The disqualification
under the 1967 breath test law can be waived only if there are
certain special reasons which the court can take into consideration. For this to be done, there must be extenuating circumstances directly connected with the commission of the offence.

Thus, special reasons were considered to apply in a case in which a motorist, who normally drank shandies, was given a drink laced with vodka without his knowledge. Similarly, a medical emergency could constitute a special reason for not being disqualified.

As the number of breath tests is running at about 50,000 a year and motoring convictions exceed a million – constituting over 64 per cent of convictions for all offences – motorists need to become more conversant with their rights under the law as it now stands. During the past months, various ambiguities in the 1967 Act have been clarified as a result of certain cases reaching the Appeal Courts. The Act can be considered in several distinct parts.

*Breath tests*
Kerbside tests may be carried out only with the officially approved device by a *uniformed* constable who has 'reasonable cause' to suspect a person of having alcohol in his blood or of having committed a moving traffic offence.

In the early days of the breath test, several motorists successfully evaded prosecution by claiming that no evidence had been produced to show that the appliance used had been approved by the Secretary of State (*Scott* v. *Baker* (1968) 132 J.P. 422, 2 ALL E.R. 998). As a result of these cases, the Stationery Office provided two forms (the Breath Test Device (Approval) (No. 1) Order, 1968 and the Breath Test Device (Approval) (No. 2) Order, 1968) to be used by the prosecution (*R.* v. *Clarke (James)* (1969) 133 J.P. 282, 1 ALL E.R. 924). It is, however, no longer necessary for these forms to be employed, as the Court of Appeal has ruled, in a case involving a motorist from Cheshire, that the prosecution need no longer prove that the 'Alcotest 80' has been approved, as it 'would arouse derision' if the law continued to demand formal proof. It has also been ruled that production of the breath test device as an exhibit at the trial is not essential (*Miller* v. *Howe* (1969) 3 ALL E.R. 451).

The specification that the constable should be in uniform has also led to cases being dismissed on a technicality. In these the constables concerned did not state in their evidence that they were in uniform at the time when the tests were given; this was considered to be an adequate reason for the magistrates to acquit the charged motorists. Another attempted defence has been made by motorists claiming the police constable was not 'in uniform' as he was not wearing his helmet at the time the test was requested. In November 1969, the High Court closed this loophole when it ruled that a policeman is still in uniform even if he is not wearing his helmet. This part of the law does not prevent a plain-clothes policeman from stopping a suspected drunken driver, but insists on the actual breath test being administered by one in uniform. One attempt to establish a loophole by a motorist who claimed that it had been hearsay for a uniformed policeman to ask him for a breath test on the basis of a request from plain-clothes policemen has been rejected by the courts and conviction allowed to stand.

The justification for requesting a breath test on the ground of 'reasonable cause' is vague enough to take in most forms of eccentric behaviour, and it places a great deal of responsibility upon the police for them to be careful in their selection of suspects. This has resulted in several cases in which the defence has successfully claimed that a 'reasonable cause' did not exist. In one case, in Wiltshire, the motorist had been stopped for driving too closely behind the vehicle being driven by the policeman. The successful defence plea was that, as this did not constitute a moving traffic offence and the constable had no reason to suspect the accused motorist of having been drinking, then there was no valid reason for making him take the breath test.

To interpret 'reasonable cause' as applying to anybody leaving a public house has led to many erroneous results and much wasted time; although one Minister of Transport has said he could see nothing wrong in the practice of police sitting outside public houses ready to pounce on anyone about to drive a car, despite the fact that the instructions for using the 'Alcotest 80' specifically state that at least twenty minutes must elapse between the last drink and the test being carried out. There are two good reasons for this rule. Firstly, the blood alcohol, and hence the corresponding breath alcohol, level is unlikely to have reached an equilibrium, so that the test result is no true indication of whether his drinking has put a suspect over the limit. Secondly, residual mouth alcohol in saliva takes about twenty minutes to disperse after drinking, and any test during this period will almost certainly produce an artificially high reading.

The question of the twenty minutes led to a test-case (*Webber* v. *Carey* (1969) 3 ALL E.R. 406) being taken to the Queen's Bench Divisional Court. This court upheld the rejection of charges against the motorist on the ground that the test carried out did not comply with the instructions, in that it was given within twenty minutes of the motorist's last drink. Because of the progressive weakening of the Road Safety Act 1967, the case of the twenty minutes in Michael P. Carey's case, just referred to, was taken to the House of Lords (*Director of Public Prosecutions* v. *Carey*, H. of L., 3 December 1969). The Lords allowed a police appeal against the original Queen's Bench Divisional Court decision and rejected the defence that the police must follow precisely the instructions issued with the breath-testing device. This decision has clarified several points. It places the onus on the motorist to notify the police if less than twenty minutes has passed since he last took alcohol, and means that it is no longer incumbent upon a policeman to establish when a motorist had his last drink. The instructions do not form an integral part of the device and the Act does not require that the breath test be carried out in strict compliance with the instructions. It is enough for the policeman to act in good faith and for him to endeavour to use the appliance correctly to achieve a true result.

As a result of successful appeals in the lower courts on the ground of an insufficient time interval, the police were advised to ensure that the test complied fully with the manufacturers' instructions supplied with each kit of 'Alcotest 80'. This normally meant devising delaying tactics by the police to keep the detained motorist waiting for the twenty minutes. As a result, additional loopholes opened up with the stopped motorist walking away from his car and therefore technically being no longer a driver, or by taking another alcoholic drink while waiting or by smoking a cigarette and thereby invalidating the test.

Included in the instructions for applying the breath test are that the 'Alcotest 80' should not be stored above 30°C. (86°F.). This has resulted in the acquittal of a motorist in a case in Lancashire in which the test was given on a breath tube which had been stored in a police car during a heat-wave. Another requirement of the test is that the plastic bag should be inflated with one continuous blow lasting between ten and twenty seconds. This has been undermined by a decision in the Scottish Appeal Court in which the judge ruled that there was no power to arrest, as a breath sample, given with two blows, gave a negative reading. In contradiction to this, another motorist, in Leicestershire, was considered to have failed to provide a breath sample as he filled the bag with nine short puffs. The prosecution successfully claimed that breath was defined as coming from the lungs and the nine puffs meant it only came from the mouth.

To be able to require a breath test in the case of *any* moving traffic offence would seem to be throwing the net very wide indeed. This means that, in theory, anyone driving at night with a faulty side-light or dead number-plate light can be asked to blow into the bag. It would be preferable for this to be restricted to drivers involved in accidents or actually charged with committing a moving traffic offence. It seems only reasonable to suggest that no test should be permitted unless there is a definite intention to charge the driver for the offence that has been the reason for having him stopped.

While the Home Office has always asserted that the police do not make tests at random, but are selective according to the law, frequent criticisms have been made that the low percentage of positive tests indicates that these have, in fact, been carried out on an *ad hoc* basis. In the first three months of the breath test from October 1967, only 40 per cent of the tests were positive. By May 1968 this figure had risen to 55 per cent and was considered by a spokesman for the Automobile Association to show a decrease in random testing and an improvement in police discrimination. The monthly figures for breath tests now show a fairly consistent pattern of 50 to 55 per cent giving positive results in any one month. Just over half of these are requested after road accidents, and the balance for moving traffic violations and for drivers believed to have been drinking.

A person refusing a kerbside breath test can be automatically arrested without a warrant. At the police station he must be asked a second time to give a breath sample before he can be asked to give a blood sample.

The penalty for refusing to give a breath sample at the road-side is a fine not exceeding £50. It is a mistake to believe that, if a driver later takes a breath test or supplies a blood sample at the police station, he cannot be fined for refusing to give the initial breath sample. In a case at Portsmouth, a driver who later supplied a blood sample was fined £5 for having refused earlier to provide a breath sample when stopped at the road-side.

In some earlier cases it was maintained that the police have no right to arrest a person under the 1967 Act after he has left his vehicle and entered his home. This point was established by several cases that went to the Appeal Court. In one case, the Criminal Appeal Court quashed the conviction on the ground that a person ceases to be a driver on entering his home and in these circumstances the breath test should not have been requested (*Campbell* v. *Tormey* (1969), 133 J.P. 267). At the same time, it was pointed out that a driver can still be charged under the 1960 Road Traffic Act if he is seen to be driving when his ability is impaired owing to drink or drugs. It has also been established that a person is still a driver even if he leaves his car, provided he does so for a purpose connected with driving, e.g. to obtain petrol (*R.* v. *Price* (1968) 1 W.L.R. 1853. C.A.).

More recently, in the case of John E. Jones of Breconshire (4 December 1969), the Appeal Court Judge, Lord Justice Sachs, stated that, 'It is not in the view of this Court the law that a motorist, merely by turning off a highway, can stultify police action and escape being required to give a breath test, when the action would otherwise be proper.' In this particular instance, the driver had been stopped after turning into his own drive, and so it can be considered as constituting a differ-ent set of circumstances from those which apply when a motorist has stopped his car, alighted, and actually entered his house.

### Blood and urine tests

Where a breath test has indicated that the driver's alcohol content is above the 80 mg. level, he is formally arrested and taken to the police station to provide a specimen of blood or urine. Failure to make a formal arrest by the policeman either taking hold of the motorist or saying 'I arrest you' has led to several charges being dismissed even when the blood alcohol levels have been shown to be well in excess of the 80 mg. limit.

The request for a blood or urine sample can be made automatically if the person has refused to give the previously requested breath sample. Refusal to supply a body fluid sample after three requests leads to automatic conviction, as though the motorist had given a sample that proved he was above the limit. Under these circumstances the only evidence required by a court is proof that the driver was in charge of a motor vehicle and had refused to supply the sample when asked.

Several well-defined steps must be taken before a driver can be charged on the basis of having failed to provide a specimen suitable for analysis. He must first be requested and have refused to supply a sample of blood. This must be followed by a request to the driver, and a refusal on his part, to supply two samples of urine within an hour. Finally, a third request, again for a blood sample, must be declined before a charge of refusing to provide a sample can be made. This whole procedure is weighted in favour of the motorist, as he progressively continues to use up alcohol from his system during the intervals between requests for samples. In practice, this means that anyone marginally over the limit when first stopped by the police will almost certainly be below the limit if no blood sample is given until the final request.

*Blood samples*

These must be taken by a medical practitioner, who must sign a certificate stating that the sample was taken with the driver's consent. As things stand, the law does not define the parts of the anatomy from which blood samples may be taken. This has provided an escape for a number of motorists who have created almost impossible situations by offering their big toe or penis as the sample area. These gaps in the law now appear to have been closed. In a case in Manchester, the magistrates ruled that a police surgeon was right in refusing to take a blood sample from a motorist's foot, and in North London a driver was found guilty of failing to supply a sample after asking the doctor to take it from his penis. The doctor in this case considered this offer to constitute a 'refusal to co-operate'. Any future law will need to be worded more precisely on this particular aspect.

Although the government leaflet on drinking and driving, issued as a guide in 1967, states that the driver can give a second breath test at the police station as part of the 1967 Act, no legal obligation exists on the police to ask for a second breath test. This leaflet also states that the driver is entitled to have his own sample to have a private analysis carried out. This right was not written into the 1967 Act, although it had previously existed under the 1962 Road Traffic Act, and it is the procedure laid down under the earlier Act that is followed by the police surgeons. All samples, whether for private or police analysis, must be placed in containers with seals on them to prevent any interference or evaporation until required for analysis. Police evidence on blood samples has been held to be inadmissible in cases in which the driver was supplied with a sample that was too small for a private analysis to be made. A similar ruling has been made in cases in which the private analysis sample has clotted or dried up in the sample tube. This is an important point, as it suggests that the driver must have the same opportunity as the police to assess the blood alcohol level; that is, the sample must be one that is capable of analysis (*Earl* v. *Roy* (1969) 2 ALL E.R. 684).

*Urine samples*
The police require two samples taken within a one-hour period. This is because the first sample is disregarded, since its main purpose is to clear the bladder completely, so enabling urine in equilibrium with the blood to be obtained for the second sample. An adequate portion of the urine sample may also be retained by the driver for a private analysis.

It is usual for the plastic ampoule containing the motorist's sample to be sealed inside an envelope. To ensure that this is not tampered with before a private analysis is carried out, both the station sergeant and the motorist sign their names across the envelope's closed flap. Even this, however, can be an insufficient precaution against fraud and the author has met one motorist who claimed to have steamed open the reverse end of the envelope and to have diluted the blood containing alcohol, taken from his arm, with fresh blood taken from his fingers.

Where police analysts and private analysts have produced conflicting results, with the former being above the prescribed limit and the latter below, the magistrates have tended, although not invariably, to find the accused not guilty because of the contradictory nature of the evidence. This confusion has arisen partly because of a failure to draw attention to the limitations of the analytical procedures and also because the samples submitted for independent analysis have sometimes been poorly sealed and have partially evaporated. It would therefore appear that a preferable procedure would be for the police to retain all the samples until a motorist has found a private analyst to deal with his sample, which could then only be obtained by the analyst directly from the police laboratories. This would prevent fraud and ensure that the sample was being kept under refrigerated conditions at all times.

In cases where a driver has been injured in an accident and taken to hospital, the police are not entitled to make any tests or take any samples without the consent of the medical practitioner in charge of the patient. The medical practitioner is entitled to refuse permission for the taking of samples in cases where he considers it could be inimitable to the treatment of the patient.

It should be emphasized that breath tests can only be applied to persons driving or in charge of motor vehicles. The Road Safety Act 1967 has no clause permitting the police to ask cyclists or pedestrians to submit to a breath test. A policeman who made a drunken cyclist take a breath test was exceeding his powers and was leaving himself open to legal proceedings.

To sum up, the law as it now stands has written into it the following safeguards for the driver:

(a) Requests for roadside breath tests can only come from a uniformed police constable.

(b) Tests must be carried out with apparatus that has been approved for this purpose by the Home Secretary.

(c) No patient in hospital can be asked to take the test without the consent of the medical practitioner in charge.

(d) A person failing to take a kerbside breath test must be given the opportunity to provide one at the police station before he can be asked to give a urine or blood sample.

(e) A blood or urine sample can only be requested if the breath test has indicated that the driver is above the prescribed limit or if he has refused to take the breath test.

(f) A blood sample can only be taken by a qualified medical

practitioner, and only then with the consent of the person concerned.

(g) A person required to supply a blood or urine sample must be warned in advance by the police constable that refusal to supply the sample may make him liable to imprisonment, a fine and disqualification. Failure to give this warning can lead to any case being dismissed in court.

(h) The person supplying a blood or urine sample is entitled, under the 1962 Act, to retain a sealed portion of the sample for a private analysis to be carried out.

Although the rights of the individual are protected by these legal requirements, it is still felt by many people that more safeguards are necessary if we are to ensure that the motorist is fairly treated under the law. Because of the loose wording in the 1967 Act and the large number of loopholes that have appeared in it, it would benefit from rewriting before further loopholes are disclosed to undermine it still further.

One important change made by the 1967 Act is that the offence of driving, or attempting to drive, with a blood alcohol level in excess of the prescribed limit has become absolute. A driver can no longer call his medical doctor to give evidence that he is sober. A detained driver can only ask for his own doctor to be called in the event of injury or illness, but not for the purpose of ascertaining his sobriety.

It is also important to emphasize that a person can still be charged under the earlier Acts for being drunk in charge. The new Act does not replace the others, but only supplements them. A motorist whose blood alcohol level was only 70 mg./100 ml. has been succesfully charged with driving under the influence of drink on the basis of the 1962 Road Traffic Act. But in such cases a motorist must be clearly told that he is likely to be charged under the earlier Acts.

Lord Chief Justice Parker, dealing with a case in which the 1967 breath test Act did not apply, has advised the police: 'Where the circumstances justify it, where impairment of a driver is reasonably suspected, the proper course for a police officer is to make it clear that the arrest is not only as a result of the new law but also under the 1962 Act.'

# CHAPTER NINE
# A Call for Accuracy

It will by now be apparent to the reader that, although the members of the medical and scientific professions have tried to establish well-defined standards of accuracy, there are still limitations to the various sampling and analytical methods which have been recommended and adopted. The scientists involved are only too conscious of these limitations, and articles in specialist journals frequently draw attention to this fact.

The law has always had this habit of over-simplifying scientific results and recommendations. Simply because the law states that the level of alcohol in the blood must be no greater than 80 mg. does not mean that this figure can be determined exactly without any possibility of inaccuracy or variation. Just as the speed shown on a car speedometer will depend upon the accuracy of that piece of machinery, so the accuracy of any scientific method will depend upon the apparatus, the chemicals and the operator. Since the law draws no attention to this aspect, it is probably fair to say that the average magistrate also remains unaware of it.

There are three sources of error which can still arise in a breath test despite the legal safeguards listed in the preceding chapter.

First, there is considerable difficulty in telling if the green coloration has reached, or passed, the mark when the test is carried out under the rather poor lighting of some streets or under a beam from a police torch. Even car headlamps are hardly an ideal spot for assessing a positive result. Because of this, and in the interests of common justice, a second breath test should *always* be made at a police station before the motorist is subjected to the indignity of supplying a blood or urine sample. In the meantime, studies should be initiated to check the extent of misreading of breath tubes that can occur under artificial light. Until this has been done, it should not be an offence to refuse to take a breath test in the street if one is given immediately afterwards at the police station.

Secondly, it is well established that opened tubes are likely to undergo the chemical change automatically if left exposed to the atmosphere for long periods. The law does not require that the breath tube is opened and fitted in the sight of the driver, and even the manufacturers' instructions for the use of the 'Alcotest 80' only caution that the indicator colour should be checked as a clear yellow. This means that, in practice, it is possible for a policeman to drive around for several hours with a prepared apparatus while watching for a suitable candidate. While this is unlikely, specific instructions should be given stating that the sealed ampoule containing the test crystals should only have its sealed ends removed under the scrutiny of the driver of the stopped vehicle.

Thirdly, the plastic bag employed in breath tests may be used up to ten times before being discarded. It is essential for it to be flattened completely after each test and before the next. Failure to do this will mean a smaller volume of breath being blown through the tube in a subsequent test and a correspondingly low breath alcohol reading. The measured volume depends, in any case, upon the capacity of the bags, which must be manufactured to within very small tolerances. A more precise form of measuring the volume would without doubt be welcome.

Such potential sources of error as these have led to considerable doubt being cast upon the accuracy of the breath tube; a complete reassessment is now essential if public confidence in the system is to be restored.

Far too much emphasis has been placed upon the absolute values obtained from analyses of blood and urine samples. This may or may not be deliberate, but if the police analysts report that a particular sample has an alcoholic content above the limit they are misleading everybody if they give just one specific figure for that level. The publication of both police and private results should be framed in one of two ways: either (a) by stating the value obtained in the analysis and indicating the limits of possible error owing to the analytical method employed; or (b) by stating the lowest possible blood alcohol level that could give a particular analytical result.

With results expressed in this form conviction can be justified when the analytical figures show that the blood alcohol level was a minimum of 81 mg./100 ml.; but would mean no charges being brought against drivers when samples analysed at 81 mg. ±5 mg., as the possible range of samples able to give this value stands as low as 76 mg.

From the kind of answers that have been given to parliamentary questions on blood tests, it is apparent that the government is not entirely happy about the way in which analytical results are expressed. Their solution has, however, been to deduct a flat rate of 6 mg. from all analytical figures and to proceed with charges if the resulting value is still above 80 mg./100 ml. This point does not appear to be all that much emphasized when results are produced in court; in any case, the authorities would be on much stronger ground if results were expressed in a more scientific manner. The 6 mg. margin of deviation at present allowed is based upon a statistical study of the degree of error that can occur. Even this is considered to be inadequate by some experts, and tolerance figures as high as 13 mg. (as in Sweden) have been suggested to ensure that due allowance is made for all circumstances.

In taking samples for analysis, several changes are needed in the present unreliable methods before anybody can have any real confidence in the results:

(a) The taking of urine samples should be stopped until the 1·33 relationship between urine and blood alcohol levels has been conclusively demonstrated and the present criticisms (see page 41) adequately answered.
(b) All blood samples should be taken by syringe from a vein, not as a few drops from the ear lobe or thumb.
(c) Samples should be sufficient to fill completely the sample containers, which should be fitted with air-tight caps and contain sufficient anti-coagulant to ensure that samples arrive at the laboratories in a usable condition.
(d) Sample containers should be secured with embossed seals to prevent any tampering being possible before analysis is carried out.

These points, which have worried many informed people since breath testing was introduced, have also been of major concern to the British Medical Association. In 1968, after the tests had been running for about a year (a sufficient time interval for results and discrepancies to be clearly identified), a special committee of the B.M.A. made a list of eleven recom-' mendations for changes in the testing procedures. So far no action has been taken by the Home Secretary upon these proposals, though they were forwarded to him.

One major point of contention felt by most motorists is over the way in which the motoring fraternity has been progressively singled out for specialist restrictive treatment during the past few years. Certainly the number of cars on the roads is increasing faster than other form of traffic; but this does not mean that only drivers of motor vehicles are involved in accidents. In fact in 1967 nearly one third of all casualties were either pedestrians or cyclists, and various researchers have shown that over 40 per cent of pedestrians killed in road accidents have quantities of blood alcohol in excess of 30 mg./100 ml. A person who has been drinking heavily can be just as much a menace to others as a pedestrian or a cyclist as he would be if a motorist.

Most drivers have had the unnerving experience of trying to avoid a drunken cyclist swerving all over the road, or of having to brake rapidly to avoid a drunk stepping off the pavement. The law on 'moving traffic violations' should apply equally to the large number of cyclists travelling without lamps, as it does to the motorist. As the law now stands, a sober motorist involved in an accident with a drunken cyclist or pedestrian can be asked to blow into the breath tube while the cause of the accident can stand by grinning, knowing that he is not obliged by law to undergo the same examination.

A great deal of resentment over the breath test originates from this preferential treatment and the law should be changed to make it possible for anyone involved in a road accident or controlling a malfunctioning vehicle to be obliged to submit to the breath test.

When the present Act is rewritten, it would be a good idea if this and all the earlier Acts could be consolidated into a single motoring Act so that motorists can be clearer about their responsibilities. As it is, the numerous Road Traffic Acts all contain special sections repealing or altering parts of earlier Acts. This may keep the legal profession happily occupied, but it adds to the worries of the average motorist.

# CHAPTER TEN
# The Future

As the realm of road safety comes within the domain of the Ministry of Transport, and the responsibility for ensuring that laws are enforced comes under the control of the Home Office, it is difficult to forecast, with any degree of accuracy, the changes likely to occur in institutions so dependent upon political vagaries. With all the science now being brought to bear upon law enforcement, there is always the possibility that the Ministry of Science and Technology will make a takeover bid for both the other ministries.

A general trend in road safety thinking does, however, seem to exist independently of the political prejudices so common in other national issues. An intention to introduce some form of breath test was obviously developing in the Ministry of Transport during the early 1960s under the then Conservative government. In all probability, the actual introduction of tests would have come about irrespective of any change in the political complexion in 1964. Already, at that time, as a result of the 1962 Road Traffic Act, a motorist could be charged if his ability to drive properly was *impaired* owing to drink or drugs; it was not necessary for him to be incapable. The same Act of Parliament also enabled the police to request a sample of blood, urine or breath for laboratory analysis, though no system for determining the alcohol content of a breath sample was adopted or recommended at that time.

Mrs Barbara Castle's name will be forever engraved in the annals of motoring as the Minister responsible for initiating breath tests in Britain, and in so doing contributing to a substantial reduction in the numbers of road casualties. It is, however, quite obvious that, while such tests are well justified, not everything in the road safety garden is rosy, and future

Ministers of Transport may need to take further steps to curb the numbers of deaths still occurring as a result of drinking.

Should the accident figures again start to show a regular increase and reach a stage where they indicate no improvement upon those existing before the 80 mg./100 ml. limit was imposed, there is every likelihood that a new 50 mg./100 ml. limit will be introduced. Recent monthly accident figures (to the end of 1969) do seem to indicate that the original effects of the breath test are wearing off; no new law would be required to bring a lower limit into force, as the present law enables the Minister to introduce any other proportions by statutory instrument. A 50 mg. limit would bring us into line with a majority of the countries which have these tests, and at least there would be more justification for this particular level than there ever was for the present one. Such a step would undoubtedly lead to further claims about vendettas against the motorist and publican, though there is little evidence that beer and spirit sales have permanently suffered under the present situation.

Although the present Minister of Transport, Mr F. Mulley, has listened to the increasing volume of criticism levelled against the loopholes in the 1967 Act, and has set up a committee to look into the matter, it may well be some considerable time before further legislation can be brought in to sort out the confusion. Until then there will certainly be further contested breath test cases to cause embarrassment to the police. The great danger is that legislation may eventually be rushed through to deal with the obvious loopholes but fail to come to grips with the wider problems mentioned in this book.

Considerable interest has been aroused by a suggestion made by the Recorder of Newbury, Mr Edward Terrell, Q.C., that the term of the automatic disqualification for driving with more than the prescribed blood alcohol level should operate on a sliding scale increasing with the blood alcohol content. The scale suggested is:

80–100 mg.: 3 months' disqualification
100–130 mg.: 6 months' disqualification
130–150 mg.: 12 months' disqualification
150–200 mg.: 2 years' disqualification

A system such as this has much to commend it, but would only be workable if a well-standardized method of expressing results could be established. The present approach of simply deducting 6 mg. and prosecuting if the result is over the limit, is obviously undesirable and would be made more so in any sliding scale, which would lead to an increase in marginal cases lying between one level and another.

There is also a distinct possibility that other more robust forms of breath-testing devices will eventually be introduced. Certainly an apparatus using automatic optical systems would be more desirable than the current visual determination, and it could, in the long run, lead to a great saving of police time if an increase in accuracy meant that more marginal cases would be eliminated at an early stage. The B.M.A. has recognized the potential in this area and is supporting the apparatus invented by Dr B. Wright of the Medical Research Council. This particular instrument suffers, in common with 'Alcotest 80', from the disadvantage that its accuracy is dependent upon the operator making a visual assessment of the colour change. An automatic meter or chart record of the result would be preferable and less subject to human error and fallibility. As a large number of different machines and devices have been developed for this purpose over the years, no apparatus should be adopted until full consideration has been given to all those available. In the interests of justice and accuracy, only the best should be good enough.

Despite all attempts at public relations, the average person remains badly informed about the methods available for studying alcohol in body fluids. If this book results in a greater dissemination of the freely available knowledge, it will have served its purpose. People have no respect for laws which they do not understand, nor for science that cloaks itself in a veil of mystery. Laws need to be written in a language which can be understood by the majority of the community, and science needs to be explained in a manner that is comprehensible to the layman. Professional groups have a habit of developing their own methods of communication which revolve around artificial languages of their own making – and then they complain when 'other people' (meaning anyone outside their particular circle) cannot understand or communicate with them. The whole idea of public relations is based upon putting across a complicated subject in a style which is easily to be understood by a majority of people. In the realm of breath and blood tests public relations have been a lamentable failure and have led to the present widespread distrust of the scientific methods involved. This state of affairs will continue until, if ever, our legislators realize that laws are made for people and not people for laws.

# Bibliography

## Books and official publications

1. A. S. Curry (ed.), *Methods of Forensic Science*, Vol. 4, Chapter 1: 'Methods of Determining Alcohol', by H. Ward-Smith, Interscience, 1965.
2. F. Lundquist (ed.), *Methods of Forensic Science*, Vol. 2, Chapter 4: 'The Application of Gas Chromatography in Forensic Science', by W. J. Cadman, Interscience, 1963.
3. Road Traffic Act 1962, H.M.S.O., 1962.
4. Road Safety Act 1967, H.M.S.O., 1967.
5. *The New Law on Drinking and Driving*, H.M.S.O., 1967.
6. *Chemical Tests for Intoxication*, Committee on Medico-legal Problems, American Medical Association, 1959.
7. *Recognition of Intoxication*, British Medical Association, 1958.
8. *The Drinking Driver*, British Medical Association, 1965.
9. P. G. M. Gregory, *The Plight of the Motorist*, Conservative Political Centre, 1968.
10. *Road Accident Statistics, 1967*, Royal Society for the Prevention of Accidents, 1967.
11. *Road Accident Statistics, 1968*, Royal Society for the Prevention of Accidents, 1968.
12. *Alcohol and Road Traffic*, British Medical Association, 1963.
13. *Research on the Effects of Alcohol and Drugs on Driver Behaviour*, O.E.C.D., 1968.
14. F. Bergel and D. R. A. Davies, in collaboration with P. Ford, *All About Drugs*, Nelson, 1970.
15. J. Cohen and B. Preston, *Causes and Prevention of Road Accidents*, Faber & Faber, 1968.

16. J. J. Leeming, *Road Accidents – Prevent or Punish*, Cassell, 1969.
17. *Research on Road Safety* (by the Road Research Laboratory), H.M.S.O., 1963.
18. *Blutalkohol*, Vols. 1–6, Steinbec, Hamburg.
19. *Medicine, Science and Law*, Vols. 1–9, Sweet & Maxwell.
20. L. G. Norman, *Road Traffic Accidents – Epidemiology, Control and Prevention*, World Health Organization, 1962.

# Articles

1. D. W. Kent-Jones and G. Taylor, 'Determination of Alcohol in Blood and Urine', *Analyst* (1954), *79*, pp. 121–136.
2. D. W. Kent-Jones, 'Interpretation of Analytical Tests for Intoxication', *Journal of the Royal Institute of Chemistry* (1967), pp. 491–500.
3. G. Chedd, 'The Hazards of a Pin-prick', *New Scientist* (1968), pp. 577–9.
4. J. P. Payne, D. W. Hill and D. G. L. Wood, 'Distribution of Ethanol Between Plasma and Erythrocytes in Whole Blood', *Nature* (1968), *217*, pp. 963–4.
5. J. P. Payne, D. V. Foster, D. W. Hill and D. G. L. Wood, 'Observations on Interpretation of Blood Alcohol Levels Derived from Analysis of Urine', *British Medical Journal* (1967), *3*, p. 819.
6. M. Day, G. G. Muir and J. Watling, 'Evaluation of "Alcotest R80" Reagent Tubes', *Nature* (1968), *219*, pp. 1051–2.
7. J. Berkebile, 'The Intoximeter', *Journal of Chemical Education* (1954), *31*, pp. 380–2.
8. M. Hellicar, 'The Year of the Breath Test', *Daily Mirror*, 27 September 1968.
9. *Road Accident Statistical Review* (Royal Society for the Prevention of Accidents), Nos. 37 and 38 (1967), 41, 44, 48, 49, 50 (1968), 60 (1969).
10. 'Breath Tests: A Year Later', *Drive* (Automobile Association), Autumn 1968.
11. D. S. Miller, J. L. Stirling and J. Yudkin, 'Effect of

Ingestion of Milk on Concentrations of Blood Alcohol', *Nature* (1966), p. 1051.

12. J. D. J. Havard, 'The Road Safety Bill, Part 1 – A Medical View', *Criminal Law Review* (1967), p. 151.

13. G. O. Jeffcoate, 'An Examination of Reports of Fatal Road Accidents in Three Police Districts from the point of View of the Effect of Alcohol', *British Journal of Addiction* (1958), *54*, p. 81.

14. G. C. Drew, W. P. Colquhoun and H. A. Long, 'Effect of Small Doses of Alcohol on a Skill Resembling Driving', *British Medical Journal* (1958), p. 993.

15. J. Cohen, E. J. Dearnaley and C. E. M. Hansel, 'The Risk Taken in Driving Under the Influence of Alcohol', *British Medical Journal* (1958), p. 1438.

16. P. Gillman, 'The Day I Was Grounded', *Sunday Times Magazine*, 12 October 1969.

17. N. Dunnett and K. J. Kimber, 'Urine-Blood Alcohol Ratio', *Journal of Forensic Science* (1968), *8*, p. 15.

18. A. S. R. Sinton, 'Examination for Sobriety', *Journal of Forensic Science* (1960), *1*, p. 21.

19. Press and Law Reports from: *The Times, Sunday Times, Daily Telegraph, Daily Express, Daily Mail, Daily Sketch* and *Daily Mirror*.

# Patents

1. R. F. Borkenstein: British Patent 821,013.
2. T. Kitagawa: British Patent 1,011,929.
3. D. Julita and J. Hayoz: British Patent 1,070,199.
4. M. Dragerwerk: German Patent 932,750.
5. M. Dragerwerk: German Patent 1,037,726.
6. L. A. Mokhov: Russian Patent 101,750.
7. R. N. Harger: U.S. Patent 2,062,785.
8. C. Ferguson: U.S. Patent 2,141,646.
9. G. C. Forrester: U.S. Patent 2,591,691.
10. R. N. Harger: U.S. Patent 2,867,511.
11. K. Grosskopf: U.S. Patent 2,939,768.
12. M. J. Luckey: U.S. Patent 3,009,786.
13. M. J. Luckey: U.S. Patent 3,223,488.
14. M. L. Moberg, E. M. Wilson and P. J. Meredith: U.S. Patent 3,338,087.

# APPENDIX A

## Chemical Tests for Alcohol

Methods available for the chemical analysis of blood, urine and breath samples can be classified into two groups. The first of these are qualitative tests: so-called because they are only used to show the existence of alcohol, but not necessarily the amount present. The second group are the quantitative tests employed to determine the amount of alcohol present within an established level of accuracy. It will be appreciated that, while a quantitative test may also be a qualitative test, the converse is not necessarily true.

The present breath test employed in Great Britain is basically a rough quantitative measure developed from a qualitative test. Because of this, its accuracy is rather limited and it is only suitable as a screening test in cases where people are either near or over the limit. Of necessity this requires a more precise study after a positive response to the tests has been obtained and is the reason for taking a blood or urine sample in such cases.

The majority of the tests employed for checking the presence and quantity of alcohol (more specifically we should refer to ethyl alcohol) are based upon the chemical reactions that it will undergo in the presence of chemical reagents known as oxidizing agents. These are chemicals which are able to supply oxygen to a system to bring about a chemical change on other substances; in this case on the ethyl alcohol.

Ethyl alcohol, the active constituent of alcoholic beverages, is a member of a group of closely related chemicals known collectively as the 'alcohols'. Also included in this group are methyl alcohol, propyl alcohol and butyl alcohol along with many others. The alcohols consist of a combination of carbon, hydrogen and oxygen atoms, expressed by the chemist in a shorthand form as:

| $CH_3OH$ | methyl alcohol |
| $CH_3CH_2OH$ | ethyl alcohol |
| $CH_3CH_2CH_2OH$ | propyl alcohol |
| $CH_3CH_2CH_2CH_2OH$ | butyl alcohol |

Thus, ethyl alcohol is the second member of a chemical series in which consecutive members differ from the previous member by one additional carbon atom and two additional hydrogen atoms.

In the chemical reactions mentioned throughout this book, attack by the oxidizing agents leads to a progressive breakdown of the structure of ethyl alcohol. Oxidation takes place in three distinct steps, depending upon the amount of oxygen supplied to the reacting system.

In the first step, a limited amount of available oxygen leads to the formation of acetaldehyde. In chemical terms this is represented by the following chemical equation:

$$CH_3CH_2OH \ + \ O \longrightarrow CH_3CHO \ + \ H_2O$$
Ethyl alcohol    Oxygen    Acetaldehyde    Water

With a larger amount of available oxygen, the oxidation proceeds further producing acetic acid, represented by a second chemical equation:

$$CH_3CHO \ + \ O \longrightarrow CH_3COOH$$
Acetaldehyde    Oxygen    Acetic acid

Under more severe reaction conditions, the acetic acid is oxidized to its maximum extent to form carbon dioxide and water; as represented in the third chemical equation:

$$CH_3COOH \ + \ 4\,O \longrightarrow 2\,CO_2 \ + \ 2\,H_2O$$
Acetic acid    Oxygen    Carbon dioxide    Water

Many chemicals are capable of supplying the oxygen required for these reactions to occur, but in practice only a few well-established systems are employed. While it is not possible in a book of this nature to discuss all the chemical methods that have been tried, there are three that stand out above all others for the extent of their application. These are:

(a) Oxidation by a solution of potassium dichromate, or related chemicals, in sulphuric acid.

(b) Oxidation by a solution of potassium permanganate in sulphuric acid.

(c) Oxidation by iodine pentoxide.

The first of these reagents, potassium dichromate, produces a yellow-orange solution when dissolved in dilute sulphuric acid. If a reactive substance such as ethyl alcohol is added to the solution, a colour change from yellow-orange to blue-green takes place. The new coloration is due to the formation of chromium sulphate in the reaction. This is the cause of the green colour that arises when alcohol is blown through the tube of the 'Alcotest 80'. Using a chemical equation, this is expressed as:

$$2\,K_2Cr_2O_7 + 8\,H_2SO_4 \longrightarrow 2\,Cr_2(SO_4)_3 + 2\,K_2SO_4 + 8\,H_2O + 6\,O$$

| Potassium dichromate | Sulphuric acid | Chromium sulphate | Potassium sulphate | Water | Oxygen |

The oxygen from this reaction is responsible for converting the ethyl alcohol to acetaldehyde and, ultimately, to acetic acid, as already described. The further conversion to carbon dioxide and water only occurs if the potassium dichromate/sulphuric acid solution is heated with the ethyl alcohol.

The intensity of the colour change that occurs in this system is a measure of the amount of alcohol that is present, and the laboratory application of the method is dependent upon using carefully measured concentrations of specially purified chemicals so that the margin of error is kept to a minimum in quantitative determinations. The first quantitative measure of ethyl alcohol by this system was carried out as long ago as 1865, and the procedure has been used and improved extensively during the past hundred years. As a result of this work, an experienced analyst can determine the amount of alcohol in a sample of blood or urine within an accuracy of $\pm 5$ per cent. Similar limits to the degree of accuracy apply to the other methods, and because of this most of the colour-change reactions tend to be used more for screening purposes than for conclusive quantitative testing.

For the acidified potassium permanganate system, the colour change ranges from the distinctive purple colour to almost colourless. This is because the oxidation of the alcohol leads to the highly coloured potassium permanganate being destroyed as it provides oxygen for the oxidation according to the following chemical equation:

$$2 \, KMnO_4 \; + \; 3 \, H_2SO_4 \longrightarrow K_2SO_4 \; + \; 2 \, MnSO_4 + 3 \, H_2O \; + \; 5 \, O$$

Potassium   Sulphuric   Potassium   Manganese   Water   Oxygen
permanganate   acid      sulphate    sulphate

Like the previously described potassium dichromate re-action, this method has also been employed in a number of different forms of apparatus for on-the-spot determinations of breath alcohol. Under laboratory conditions, its level of accuracy is comparable to the previous method; the process is often used in other chemical studies of oxidation reactions.

The use of iodine pentoxide for the determination of ethyl alcohol differs from the other two methods as the chemical reagent is a colourless substance. Oxidation of the alcohol causes a release of free iodine that is measured by means of the formation of a blue colour with a solution of starch and potassium iodide. In this process the ethyl alcohol is fully converted through all three oxidation stages to carbon dioxide and water, as shown in the equation:

$$5 \, C_2H_5OH \; + \; 6 \, I_2O_5 \longrightarrow 10 CO_2 \; + \; 15 \, H_2O \; + \; 6 \, I_2$$

Ethyl    Iodine      Carbon    Water   Iodine
alcohol  pentoxide   dioxide

The amount of iodine produced, and hence the intensity of the blue colour, is directly related to the quantity of alcohol in the sample. This method of determination was one of the earliest employed for on-the-spot quantitative measures for breath alcohol in the U.S. It is no longer used as a laboratory procedure owing to the difficulties of maintaining a high level of accuracy.

It will be obvious that the accuracy of colour reactions depends upon many factors including the absence of other compounds likely to be oxidized by the reagents. The quantitative value of these reactions only exists if the analyst first removes any substances likely to interfere with the test. This can usually be achieved with a laboratory procedure, but is not likely to be entirely possible in roadside tests.

Many public analysts have discontinued using the above reactions for accurate determinations of the ethyl alcohol in blood and urine samples submitted to them. Instead, they resort to the technique of gas-liquid chromatography, described in detail in Chapter 7, in which all volatile substances present in the samples can be separated from each other and individually determined. The colour reactions are still employed in several ways in portable forms of apparatus used for kerbside tests of breath alcohol in the U.S. For these purposes the potassium dichromate and potassium permanganate systems still figure prominently.

# APPENDIX B

Analysts Prepared to Undertake Private Analyses of Samples for Drivers Charged with Driving with more than the Prescribed Limit of Alcohol in their Blood

The following list is published by kind permission of the Royal Institute of Chemistry, to whom the author would like to express his appreciation for their help and co-operation. As lists tend to become dated, the one below having been amended to November 1969, readers are advised to contact the Royal Institute of Chemistry, 30 Russell Square, London w.c.1, if they require a current copy of the list.

Practices are listed alphabetically by towns in six regions. The regions for this purpose are:

     England (North)
     England (Midlands)
     England (South)
     Northern Ireland
     Scotland
     Wales

Practices with facilities for carrying out gas-liquid chromatography are indicated by an asterisk *.

## ENGLAND (North)

F. W. M. Jaffe, b.sc., f.r.i.c.
     Richardson & Jaffe, 4 Claremont, Bradford 7, Yorks. (Tel. Bradford 24045)

*R. Fawcett, f.r.i.c.
     Public Analyst's Laboratory, Town Hall, Burnley, Lancs. (Tel. Burnley 25011, ext. 292)

*J. G. Sherratt, B.SC., F.R.I.C.,
and R. Sinar, B.PHARM., B.SC., F.R.I.C.
Ruddock & Sherratt, 30 Watergate Street, Chester. (Tel.
Chester 21505/6)

R. Mallinder, B.SC., F.R.I.C.
H. T. Lea & Mallinder, The Borough Laboratory, National
Provincial Bank Chambers, Halifax, Yorks. (Tel. Halifax
52826)

*R. T. Hunter, B.SC., F.R.I.C.
City Laboratories, 184 High Street, Kingston-upon-Hull.
(Tel. Kingston-upon-Hull 27847)

*R. A. Dalley, F.R.I.C.
City Analyst's Laboratory, Market Buildings, Vicar Lane,
Leeds 1. (Tel. Leeds 30211)

J. S. Merry, M.INST.F., F.R.I.C.
18 Cook Street, Liverpool 2. (Tel. Liverpool Central 3860)

*T. Harris, F.P.S., F.R.I.C.
Manchester Analytical Laboratories, 26 Corporation Street,
Manchester 4. (Tel. Manchester Blackfriars 0245)

*W. Gordon Carey, F.R.I.C.
J. & H. S. Pattison, Public Analyst's Laboratories, 10 Dean
Street, Newcastle-upon-Tyne NE1 1PG. (Tel. Newcastle
24806)

*Dr D. Blake, B.SC., A.R.I.C.
International Research and Development Ltd, Fossway,
Newcastle-upon-Tyne NE6 1PG. (Tel. Newcastle 650411)

A. C. Bushnell, F.R.I.C.
County Laboratory, County Hall, Preston PR1 8XN. (Tel.
Preston 54868, ext. 355)

*G. H. Baker, A.M.INST.P., F.R.I.C.
Melling & Ardern, 451 Lower Broughton Road, Salford 7,
Lancs. (Tel. Broughton 1822)

H. Childs, B.SC., F.R.I.C.
A. H. Allen & Partners, Public Analyst's Laboratory, 67
Surrey Street, Sheffield S1 2LH. (Tel. Sheffield 21687)

*ENGLAND (Midlands)*

\*R. K. Chalmers, B.SC., F.R.I.C.,
and C. N. Grange, B.SC., F.R.I.C.
 Bostock, Hill & Rigby, 37–39 Birchfield Road, Birmingham
 19. (Tel. Birmingham 554 2284)

\*W. M. Lewis, F.R.I.C.
 City Laboratory Service, Shortley Road, Coventry. (Tel.
 Coventry 25703)

\*E. R. Pike, B.SC., M.P.S., F.R.I.C.
 Analyst's Laboratory, Fillingate, Wanlip, Leicester LE7 8PF.
 (Tel. Leicester 813371)

Dr E. C. Wood, A.R.C.S., F.R.I.C.
 Lincolne, Sutton & Wood Ltd, Clarence House, 8 Clarence
 Road, Norwich NOR 29T. (Tel. Norwich 24555)

\*R. S. Hatfull, F.R.I.C., F.R.S.H.
 County Chemical Laboratories, County Buildings, Martin
 Street, Stafford. (Tel. Stafford 3121, ext. 13)

\*W. E. Jones, M.SC., F.R.I.C.
 County Laboratories, County Buildings, Worcester. (Tel.
 Worcester 23400)

*ENGLAND (South)*

\*Dr G. V. James, M.B.E., M.SC., F.R.I.C.
 Cook & Barke, 8 Worrall Road, Bristol 8. (Tel. Bristol
 30979)

\*Dr C. V. Reynolds, B.SC., F.R.I.C.
 Public Analyst's Laboratories, 1 Barnfield Crescent, Exeter,
 Devon. (Tel. Exeter 72836)

\*H. C. MacFarlane, A.R.T.C.S., F.R.I.C.
 Harrison & Self, Moss Lane, Godalming, Surrey. (Tel.
 Godalming 3122)

T. E. Rymer, F.R.I.C.
 Rymer & Redman, Analytical Laboratory, 1 Offham Road,
 Lewes, Sussex. (Tel. Lewes 4534)

*J. H. Shelton, F.R.I.C.
Leo Taylor & Lucke, Bedford House, Wheler Street, London
E.I. (Tel. 01–247–9260)

*J. Grant, M.SC., PH.D., F.R.I.C. and C. H. Robins, B.SC., F.R.I.C.
Hehner & Cox Ltd, 107 Fenchurch Street, London E.C.3.
(Tel. 01–488–3538)

*Dr J. H. Hamence, M.SC., F.R.I.C.
Dr Bernard Dyer & Partners (1948) Ltd, Peek House, 20
Eastcheap, London E.C.3. (Tel. Mansion House 6254)

*Dr. R. F. Milton, B.SC., M.I.BIOL., F.R.I.C.
11 Park Square West, Regent's Park, London N.W.I.
(Tel. 01–935–6559)

Dr A. J. Amos, O.B.E., B.SC., F.R.I.C.,
and Dr J. F. Herringshaw, B.SC., A.R.C.S., D.I.C., F.R.I.C.,
D. W. Kent-Jones & A. J. Amos, The Laboratories,
Dudden Hill Lane, Willesden, London N.W.10.
(Tel. 01–450–7877/9)

*D. D. Moir, M.SC., F.R.I.C., and J. A. Palgrave, B.SC., F.R.I.C.
16 Southwark Street, London S.E.I. (Tel. 01–407–2067)

D. G. Forbes, B.SC., M.CHEM.A., F.R.I.C.
325 Kennington Road, London S.E.11. (Tel. 01–735–1406)

J. H. E. Marshall, M.A., F.R.I.C.
South Eastern Laboratory, 7 Wigtown Place, London S.E.11.
(Tel. 01–735–3756)

Dr G. A. Rose, M.A., D.M., F.R.I.C., M.C.PATH.
Central Pathology Laboratories, 36 Queen Anne Street,
London W1M 9LB. (Tel. 01–580–3744)

*R. C. Spalding, M.A., F.R.I.C.
County Analyst, County Analytical Laboratory, County
Hall, Maidstone, Kent. (Tel. Maidstone 54321)

*G. B. Thackray, B.SC., F.R.I.C.
Public Analyst's Laboratory, Trafalgar Place, Clive Road,
Portsmouth, Hants. (Tel. Portsmouth 23641)

*F. A. Lyne, B.SC., F.R.I.C., and J. A. Radley, M.SC., F.R.I.C.
J. A. Radley (Laboratories) Ltd, 220–222 Elgar Road,
Reading, Berks. (Tel. Reading 82428/9)

Dr F. D. M. Hocking, M.SC., F.R.I.C.
Strathhaven, Carlyon Bay, St Austell, Cornwall.
(Tel. Par 2470)

*H. Dedicoat, F.R.I.C.
City Analyst's Laboratory, 29 Cobden Avenue, Southampton. (Tel. Southampton 55826)

*Miss J. D. Peden, B.SC., F.R.I.C.
County Laboratory, County Hall, Taunton, Somerset. (Tel. Taunton 3451)

## NORTHERN IRELAND

Dr. H. K. Lawton, B.SC., F.R.I.C.
Hawthorne & Lawton, Room 74, 16 Donegall Square South, Belfast BT1 5JJ. (Tel. Belfast 21691)

## SCOTLAND

*T. M. Clark, O.B.E., B.SC., F.R.I.C.
Regional Laboratory, City Hospital, Aberdeen. (Tel. Aberdeen 22242)

*R. S. Nicholson, F.R.I.C.
Public Analyst's Laboratory, 140 Perth Road, Dundee. (Tel. 25475)

J. M. Malcolm, F.R.I.C., J. B. McKean, F.R.I.C., and
J. W. Gray, A.M.INST.F., F.R.I.C.
R. R. Tatlock & Thompson, 156 Bath Street, Glasgow C.2. (Tel. Glasgow Douglas 0491)

*A. C. Wilson, F.R.I.C.
County Chemical Laboratory, Backford Street, Hamilton, Lanarks. (Tel. Hamilton 21100, ext. 568)

*F. N. Woodward, C.B.E., B.SC., F.R.I.C.
Arthur D. Little Research Institute, Inveresk Gate, Musselburgh, Midlothian. (Tel. Musselburgh 2434)

## WALES

*L. E. Coles, B.PHARM., PH.D., F.P.S., F.R.I.C., M.PH.A.
Glamorgan County Public Health Laboratory,

Institute of Preventive Medicine, The Parade, Cardiff.
(Tel. Cardiff 28033, ext. 496)

*A. R. Phillips, B.SC., F.R.I.C.
City Analyst's Laboratory, Crofts Street, Cardiff. (Tel.
Cardiff 31033, ext. 536 or 451)

*D. C. Jenkins, M.SC., D.I.C., F.R.I.C.
Herbert J. Evans & Partners, Public Analyst's Laboratory,
Bank Lane, Carmarthen. (Tel. Carmarthen 7536)

*A. S. Minton, F.INST.F., A.I.MAR.E., F.R.I.C.
Treharne & Davies Ltd, Merton House, Bute Crescent,
Cardiff. (Tel. Cardiff 24158)

*G. V. James, M.B.E., M.SC., F.R.I.C.
G. Rudd Thompson & Partners, 69 Dock Street, Newport,
Monmouthshire. (Tel. Newport 63035)

# Index

biochemical method of analysis, 44, 51
bladder, 11
blood alcohol: accidents and, 17, 19 *fig.* 1; levels of, 10, 34; limit of 80 mg./100 ml., 3, 52; reduction of concentration, 15; relationship with breath, 37; with urine figures, 11
blood plasma, 11
  samples: 11, 41, 47, 49, 60, 74; disinfectant for, 42; errors in, 42; and urine, 58, 61; from vein, 65
  tests, Parliamentary questions on, 65
blue coloration, 35
body tissues, alcohol in, 9
Bogen, Dr, 3
brain, rapid effect of alcohol on, 9
Bratislava, Czechoslovakia, 18
'Breathalyser', xii, 5, 25–31, 27 *fig.* 2; *see also* 'Alcotest 80'
*Breathalyzer*, 36, 37 *fig.* 6
breath-testing apparatus, other forms of, 32–9
breath-tube, modified forms of, 30–1
British Medical Association (B.M.A.), x, 3, 4, 13, 14, 15, 44, 66, 69
*British Medical Journal*, 41
British Standard Time, 23
butanol, 50

capillary blood, 11, 42
carbon dioxide, 12, 33, 34, 75, 76

Carey, Michael P., test case of, 56
cases, 52–3, 56, 58
casualty figures, 21–3, 66
Cavett micro-method, 45 *fig.* 8, 46, 47
charcoal/kaolin pills, 15
Chedd, Graham, 41
Chemical Society Library, x
chromic acid on silica particles, 37
chromium sulphate (green), 36, 76
  trioxide and sulphuric acid on silica particles, 30
colour change reactions, 26, 27, 28, 36, 37; colourless to blue, 77; purple to colourless, 33, 76; yellow-orange to blue-green, 76
concentration of blood alcohol, 36; reduction of, 15
constable in uniform, 54, 61
consumption of alcohol, 10–11, control of, 2
conversion factor, urine/blood, 40–1
conviction, automatic, 52, 59
co-ordination, deterioration of, 6, 7
cost of accidents to the nation, 20
Criminal Appeal, Court of, 58
Criminal Justice Act, 1925, 2
cyclists, no breath test for, 61, 66
Czechoslovakia, 18; legislation in, 6

deaths and injuries, grouping of, 21